# Operative Techniques in Coronary Artery Bypass Surgery

Alexander Albert
Alexander Assmann
Anna Kathrin Assmann
Hug Aubin • Artur Lichtenberg
Editors

# Operative Techniques in Coronary Artery Bypass Surgery

## An Illustrated Guide to Personalized Therapy

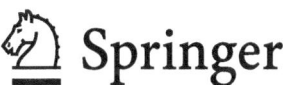 Springer

*Editors*
Alexander Albert
Medical Director
Clinic of Dortmund gGmbH -
Clinic for Heart Surgery
Beurhausstraße
Germany

Anna Kathrin Assmann
Department of Cardiac Surgery
University Hospital Düsseldorf
Düsseldorf, Nordrhein-Westfalen
Germany

Artur Lichtenberg
Department of Cardiac Surgery
University Hospital Düsseldorf
Düsseldorf, Nordrhein-Westfalen
Germany

Alexander Assmann
Department of Cardiac Surgery
University Hospital Düsseldorf
Düsseldorf, Nordrhein-Westfalen
Germany

Hug Aubin
Department of Cardiac Surgery
University Hospital Düsseldorf
Düsseldorf, Nordrhein-Westfalen
Germany

ISBN 978-3-030-48496-5          ISBN 978-3-030-48497-2    (eBook)
https://doi.org/10.1007/978-3-030-48497-2

This Springer imprint is published by the registered company Springer Nature Switzerland AG
The registered company address is: Gewerbestrasse 11, 6330 Cham, Switzerland

# Foreword

The surgical myocardial revascularization has proven to be a long-lasting therapy against myocardial ischemia and its consequences such as infarct and death. The surgical trauma related to this approach has been associated with damage to the physical and mental integrity of the patient, sometimes even neurological trauma and early lethal risk. Medical professionals have accepted this and compared themselves against reported national or international databases, but patients and society disagree and prefer alternatives with reduced early risk and visible loss of physical integrity, even at the cost of late benefit. It is therefore of utmost importance not to consider the current CABG approach as "good enough" but to reengineer constantly its process toward an annihilation of risk and an optimization of late success.

Over half a century of its availability, a few surgeons and centers were able to adapt their surgical approach to the evidence, the science of learning, the science of early and late process management and monitoring. Possible risk-reducing approaches as off-pump surgery, no-touch aorta as well as minimally invasive approaches but also early and late benefit-increasing approaches as complete arterial revascularization have not become the daily routine. Simulation training on low-fidelity modeling, OSATS-based assessments, and online mobile educational workplaces have proven to be lasting game-changers in preparing younger surgeons for the realities of a surgical theater. In my personal experience, around 6000 surgeons worldwide have been through such an educational pathway in our "My Virtual Surgery" project.

The authors of this book propose in an illustrative way how a traditional medium, such as a book, can become a complete repository of the spectrum of approaches and processes. This guide is based on the daily processes of the team surrounding Alexander Albert and Artur Lichtenberg, their previous mentors, and the patients. The strength of this guide is that it presents possibly competing surgical concepts. These concepts are placed in the perspective of the patient's variability, risk profile, anatomy, and obviously and most importantly the patient's own expectations. Every patient is different; therefore, John W. Kirklin (Mayo Clinic), Eugene H. Blackstone (Cleveland Clinic), and I developed a scientific approach toward personalized therapy in bypass surgery in the form of "patient-specific prediction" 30 years ago. The authors implemented this concept and used pragmatic checklists that lead toward flowcharts directing the decisions of the multidisciplinary teams.

Alexander Albert has been my mentor and guide in studying the science of learning and how it could impact surgical proctoring, in addition to process management toward an optimization of the surgical result. We shared a common interest in large datasets as well as mathematical modeling, while I had the privilege of guiding him toward expertise at a global level in OPCAB techniques. All these concepts are apparent or hidden in a subliminal way in this illustrated guide.

Each possible surgical strategy is deconstructed in teachable components, described step-by-step. The anastomosis technique in very reduced airspace, a mandatory skill in OPCAB and lesser invasive approach, is well described. Off-pump CABG, as any surgical process, makes only sense if it is performed after extensive simulation training and following the strictest possible standard operating procedures, not allowing the slightest drift in temperature, and avoiding, where possible, even a single extrasystole. All these at the benefit of the risk/benefit balance for the patient.

It was an extreme privilege to write the foreword of this illustrated guide to personalized therapy in CABG by Alexander Albert, Alexander Assmann and colleagues. Please enjoy and share this brilliant work.

April 21, 2020                                         Paul Sergeant, MD, PhD

# Contents

# About the Editors

**Alexander Albert, MD**
is a professor of cardiac surgery and the current director of the Department of Cardiovascular Surgery at the Klinikum Dortmund, Germany. Early in his career, professor Albert was strongly influenced by the school of Professor Paul Sergeant in Belgium. He has an internationally recognized experience in aortic no-touch off-pump (anaortic OPCAB) and minimally invasive bypass surgery (MICS-CABG). His major focus of clinical and scholarly activities lies in the development and design of individualized surgical therapy for patients with coronary artery disease. Professor Albert draws on wide experience in several managerial positions, creating and implementing new departmental processes. Additionally, he has been the head of the Medtronic International Training Center for Anaortic OPCAB and MICS-CABG since its establishment in 2010 at the University of Düsseldorf and currently at the Klinikum Dortmund. Professor Albert is involved in a collaborative effort with international experts, for example, as a faculty member in the Oxford Masterclass of Heart Surgery led by Professor David Taggart.

**Alexander Assmann, MD**
(Priv.-Doz. Dr. med.) is an attending cardiac surgeon and head of the Coronary Surgery program at the University Hospital Düsseldorf. Assmann is specialized in minimally invasive and off-pump coronary surgery and clinical proctoring for endoscopic vessel preparations. Assmann is an expert

in cardiovascular biomaterials engineering with multiple original articles and scientific awards.

**Anna Kathrin Assmann, MD**
(Dr. med.) did academic studies in human medicine at the RWTH Aachen University (2007–2013). Assmann has been a resident in cardiothoracic and pediatric cardiac surgery in the University Hospital Aachen (2014–2016) and in the University Department of Cardiac Surgery in Düsseldorf since 2016. Assmann has been a clinical proctor for endoscopic vessel preparations since 2017. Assmann's research focuses on translational cardiovascular bioimplant research.

**Hug Aubin, MD**
is an attending cardiac surgeon at the Department of Cardiac Surgery of the University Hospital Düsseldorf and head of the Mechanical Circulatory Support program. Aubin is interested in all types of minimally invasive cardiac surgery.

**Artur Lichtenberg, MD**
is the Director of the Department of Cardiac Surgery of the Heinrich-Heine-University Düsseldorf. He has been head of the Department of Cardiothoracic Surgery of the University Hospital Jena (2009) and Vice Head of the Department of Cardiac Surgery at the University Hospital Heidelberg (2006–2009). He has extensive experience in all types of CABG, performing minimally invasive CABG (MIDCAB) since as early as 1998 while training in Hannover under Prof. Haverich. He is a known expert on MIC surgery and has authored a multitude of scientific and clinical publications.

# About the Authors

**Piroze M. Davierwala**
is the lead senior consultant and director of coronary bypass surgery at the Leipzig Heart Center in Germany. He was born and raised in India, and then he attended medical school and trained in general surgery at the University of Pune, India. He pursued residency in cardiac surgery at the University of Mumbai, India. After that, he pursued fellowship training in Toronto, Canada. He went back to India and worked for two years in Pune, India. He had the chance to operate on a large number of patients in India, which made him one of the fine surgeons in cardiovascular surgery. Currently, he is working at the Leipzig Heart Center since 2009. His clinical research interests include minimally invasive valvular and coronary artery bypass surgery as well as complex reconstructive surgery for endocarditis. He has established a technique of multivessel minimally invasive coronary surgery with bilateral internal thoracic arteries without robotic or endoscopic assistance at his institute. He has published many articles in numerous peer-reviewed international journals as well as several book chapters in cardiac surgery.

**Mateo Marin-Cuartas**
graduated in medicine at the CES University in Medellin, Colombia. He is cardiac surgery resident at the Leipzig Heart Center in Leipzig, Germany as well as postdoctoral research fellow at the Cardiothoracic Surgery Department from the Stanford University School of Medicine in Stanford, California. His doctoral degree was awarded by the Leipzig University School of Medicine for his work on functional

mitral regurgitation. His research interests focus on the surgical and interventional pathology of the mitral valve, structural heart disease, and surgical coronary revascularization.

# About the Foreword Writer

**Paul Sergeant**
is a prominent professor of cardiac surgery, a scholar in CABG research, and one of the pioneers in off-pump coronary artery surgery. He is known for his skillful performance in the operating room and has helped train countless young colleagues to become outstanding surgeons. Not only in the operating room but also virtually he does help thousands of surgeons worldwide. His most recent worldwide project is called "My Virtual Surgery." With live webinars and online simulation courses and around 5500 participants from over 150 countries, "My Virtual Surgery" is one of the largest online courses for cardiac surgeons. In his training, he applies the theory of learning and the objective structured assessment of technical skills (OSATS). He became president of European Association for Cardio-Thoracic Surgery (EACTS) and was a founder and a president of The Cardiothoracic Surgery Network (CTSnet).

# Chapter 1
# Introduction

**A. Albert, A. Assmann, and A. K. Assmann**

Robust evidence has been growing that coronary artery bypass grafting (CABG) improves the outcome of patients with stable angina pectoris or silent ischemia, particularly in case of multivessel coronary disease, left main stenosis, proximal left anterior descending artery (LAD) stenosis, large ischemic area, single remaining patent coronary artery with stenosis >50%, or hemodynamically significant stenosis in the presence of angina pectoris or angina equivalent with insufficient response to optimized medical therapy. Compared to medical treatment, CABG decreases the risk of death and myocardial infarction in patients with stable coronary artery disease [1, 2].

There is general consensus that the choice of the revascularization strategy is a matter for multidisciplinary heart

A. Albert (✉)
Clinic of Dortmund gGmbH - Clinic for Heart Surgery,
Beurhausstraße, Germany
e-mail: alexander.albert@klinikumdo.de

A. Assmann · A. K. Assmann
Department of Cardiac Surgery, University Hospital Düsseldorf,
Düsseldorf, Nordrhein-Westfalen, Germany
e-mail: alexander.assmann@med.uni-duesseldorf.de; annakathrin.assmann@med.uni-duesseldorf.de

© Springer Nature Switzerland AG 2021    1
A. Albert et al. (eds.), *Operative Techniques in Coronary Artery Bypass Surgery*,
https://doi.org/10.1007/978-3-030-48497-2_1

teams, considering the patient's wish. After thorough explanation, the patient should have enough time to balance the short-term procedure-related and long-term risks and benefits of the different strategies, such as survival, potential need for subsequent re-intervention, need for prevention measures, relief from angina, quality of life, and uncertainties associated with the different strategies. Important aspects for decision making are coronary pathology (e.g. Syntax score, degree and localization of stenoses), hemodynamics (e.g. left and right systolic and diastolic cardiac function) and the pattern of comorbidities (e.g. diabetes mellitus, aortic atherosclerosis).

Daily routine shows that the option for minimally invasive coronary surgery (MICS) approaches enhances the patients' tendency towards surgical revascularization. Additionally, complete anatomical revascularization with arterial grafts, aiming at improved long-term bypass patency, may be an important argument for the decision between CABG and percutaneous coronary intervention (PCI). However, the evidence for these recommendations is still low (class IIa or IIb, level B according to the 2018 ESC/EACTS guidelines on myocardial revascularization [1]). Furthermore, there is no ideal strategy that combines optimal long-term outcome (totally arterial revascularization, complete anatomical revascularization, consideration of competitive flow phenomena) and the patients' wish for MICS.

Therefore, it is crucial to develop personalized concepts for each coronary patient, taking into account particularly age, coronary pathology, cardiac function, co-morbidities and psychological aspects. The structure of the present book reflects the core steps for decision making in CABG, and thus provides a step-by-step guide to determine an optimized strategy for each patient:

- *Strategical considerations*: In the first part of this book, the key concepts of CABG and their evidence from the literature are presented. It is defined, which techniques contribute to operative risk minimization, long-term outcome improvement, accelerated rehabilitation and enhanced quality of life. Furthermore, it is discussed for which patients the different strategies should be considered.

- *Operative techniques*: In the second part of this book, technical elements of CABG are described and illustrated step-by-step, so that a modular system is created from which specific elements can be chosen to develop personalized operative strategies. This chapter is focused on techniques the clinical establishment of which frequently causes issues, such as in off-pump coronary artery bypass grafting (OPCAB), totally arterial revascularization with bilateral internal thoracic arteries (BITA), and particularly MICS. Since expertise in off-pump techniques is a requirement for all MICS approaches, such as minimally invasive direct coronary artery bypass grafting (MIDCAB) or multivessel (MV-)MICS, and thus is indispensable for personalized CABG, the OPCAB elements are presented in detail.

- *Prototype patients*: In the third part of this book, the most frequent types of CABG are presented, and prototype patient profiles are assigned.

MICS is an evolving part of modern CABG. As MICS approaches have not yet been established in the majority of cardiosurgical centres, the present book additionally includes a separate chapter on MICS-CABG, particularly focusing on the techniques required for MV-MICS with BITA grafting.

Several presented aspects for the decision on CABG strategies and technical elements are not only based on robust evidence, but also reflect our personal experience, and therefore should be understood as recommendations and not as guideline. Our expertise has been shaped by intensive long-time experience in the broad spectrum of CABG, by our educational tasks in OPCAB, MICS and endoscopic surgery, particularly as international training centre, and by reorganization of coronary surgery programs towards OPCAB and MICS in large volume heart centres. Furthermore, personal exchange with renowned as well as less known experts in CABG is essential for us. According to this communication, we have got the impression that, despite the extensive variety of possible combinations of technical elements, several specific concepts have been established or are close to establishment, since they conform to clinical evidence and patients' wish as well as ergonomic and organizational considerations. In our experience, the prototypes presented in this book cover the vast majority of coronary surgical patients. Rare scenarios, such as gastroepiploic artery grafting or jump grafts connected by coronary artery segments [3], have been omitted.

We envision that the present book guides cardiac surgeons to become acquainted with the complete modern spectrum of CABG, in order to make personalized strategies accessible to all patients. Furthermore, we strive to inform cardiologists and patients on the potential of modern coronary bypass surgery, so that joint discussion and decision on the optimal treatment concept further improves patient care.

## References

1. Neumann FJ, Sousa-Uva M, Ahlsson A, et al. 2018 ESC/EACTS guidelines on myocardial revascularization. Eur Heart J. 2019;40:87–165.
2. Windecker S, Stortecky S, Stefanini GG, et al. Revascularisation versus medical treatment in patients with stable coronary artery disease: network meta-analysis. BMJ. 2014;348:g3859.
3. Taggart DP. How I deploy arterial grafts. Ann Cardiothorac Surg. 2018;7:690–7.

# Chapter 2
## Strategical Considerations and Key Concepts

**A. Albert, A. Assmann, and A. K. Assmann**

In contrast to detailed international guidelines concerning surgical versus interventional strategies, there is sparse evidence on the impact of different surgical approaches and techniques. According to the 2018 ESC/EACTS guidelines on myocardial revascularization, the core elements for a successful bypass operation are as follows: the complete anatomical revascularization (class I, level B) as well as the differentiated use of arterial bypass grafts (class I, level B). For the perioperative risk reduction, off-pump (class IIa, level B, or class I, level B in patients with significant aortic atherosclerosis) or even aortic no-touch (class I, level B) techniques are of importance. Minimally invasive approaches without sternotomy should be considered especially for patients with high

A. Albert (✉)
Clinic of Dortmund gGmbH - Clinic for Heart Surgery,
Beurhausstraße, Germany
e-mail: alexander.albert@klinikumdo.de

A. Assmann · A. K. Assmann
Department of Cardiac Surgery, University Hospital Düsseldorf,
Düsseldorf, Nordrhein-Westfalen, Germany
e-mail: alexander.assmann@med.uni-duesseldorf.de; annakathrin.
assmann@med.uni-duesseldorf.de

© Springer Nature Switzerland AG 2021
A. Albert et al. (eds.), *Operative Techniques in Coronary
Artery Bypass Surgery*,
https://doi.org/10.1007/978-3-030-48497-2_2

risk of sternal wound infection or in the context of hybrid procedures (class IIa or IIb, level B) [1].

Derived from available evidence, there are four crucial strategies aiming at…

1. optimization of the long-term outcome:

   (a) Complete anatomical revascularization: improves freedom from angina pectoris, long-lasting protection from myocardial infarction and survival.

   (b) Differentiated use of arterial grafts: the radial artery (RA) as well as BITA show a lower probability of atherosclerotic degeneration and therefore lower occlusion rates in the long term in contrast to saphenous veins (SV). However, arterial grafts tend to develop dysfunctions in case of high competitive flow via native vessels so that SV should be preferred in such cases. New preparation and stabilization techniques to protect the SV performance have ameliorated the vein bypass durability.

2. reduction of the operative risk:

   (c) Aortic no-touch technique: in order to reduce neurological complications due to atherosclerotic embolism from the aorta, epiaortic ultrasound should be used to detect plaques in the aorta. If aortic manipulation cannot be completely avoided, ultrasound imaging reveals areas for safe manipulation or even cannulation.

3. minimization of the surgical trauma and accelerated recovery:

   (d) MICS via left or right anterolateral thoracotomy allows for single- or multivessel bypasses without the necessity of a sternotomy. For MICS approaches, off-pump techniques are essential. In this context, surgical expertise is the most important factor regarding outcome.

The decision for a MICS operation depends on further considerations: an ideal combination of all aspects of modern bypass surgery and a MICS approach does not exist. However, for each patient, the best possible approach should be figured out by an optimal combination of the diverse existing techniques. Characteristics such as age, risk constellation, coronary status and anatomy are the most important factors to develop the best surgical approach.

As a matter of course, it is a precondition that the surgical team has expert skills in all conducted techniques, particularly in case of OPCAB. While observational studies report a 43% lower short-term mortality for OPCAB [2], it has been shown that surgeons unexperienced in the field of off-pump surgery did not reduce the risk of neurological complications, but quite the contrary occurred. More neurological complications were noted as well as poor bypass quality with a higher rate of MACCE (major adverse cardiac and cerebrovascular events) in the long term [3]. The following parameters are considered to be indicators for low quality OPCAB: a higher rate of conversion (>10%) [4], a low volume centre (<164 patients per year) or low volume surgeons (<48 patients per year) [5].

With an experienced off-pump surgeon and an experienced team, there will be no disadvantage in the long-term outcome [6]. Already in 2004, Puskas et al. demonstrated that OPCAB is as accurate and efficient as on-pump surgery [7]. On the other hand, only with the possibility of OPCAB, an individualized therapy concept can be achieved for each patient, since off-pump techniques are essential for MICS and no-touch surgery (Fig. 2.1).

While many patients can be sufficiently treated with either on- or off-pump approaches, and some patients require off-pump and MICS, there are also patients who require specifically on-pump CABG. In particular, emergency patients with severe acute myocardial ischemia and/or hemodynamic instability may not be eligible for off-pump CABG. In these cases, hemodynamic stabilization by CPB (cardiopulmonary bypass) initiation and early myocardial protection by cardioplegic arrest can be advantageous.

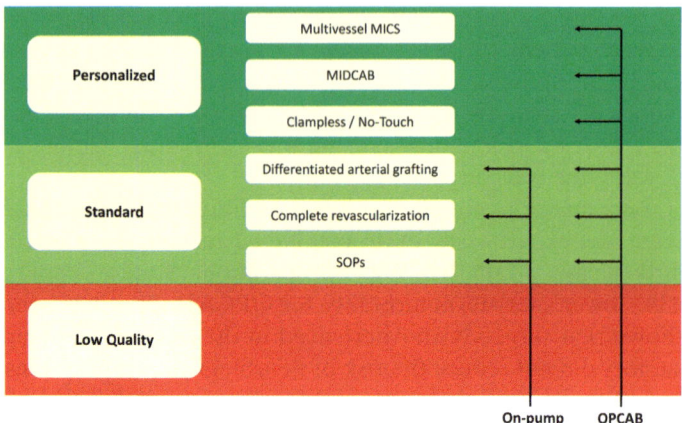

FIGURE 2.1 Strategical potential of on-pump and off-pump surgery. While on-pump surgery allows for good standard care in many patients, optimized personalized therapies for each patient require the option of MICS and avoidance of aortic manipulation. *MICS* Minimally invasive coronary surgery, *MIDCAB* Minimally invasive direct coronary artery bypass grafting, *OPCAB* Off-pump coronary artery bypass grafting, *SOPs* Standard operating procedures

In the first part of this book, a detailed description of the different surgical approaches is provided, with emphasis on technical aspects including their advantages and disadvantages.

## 2.1    Bypass Impact

The gold standard for surgical revascularization is the complete anatomical revascularization, which targets all relevant stenoses of ≥50% (estimation based on angiography) of vessels with a diameter of ≥1.5 mm [1].

Already early studies have shown the impact of incomplete revascularization on the outcome after CABG [8]. Garcia et al. demonstrated in a meta-analysis comparing complete with incomplete revascularization in patients with multivessel disease undergoing CABG or PCI that complete revascularization was associated with lower morbidity and mortality [9]. Only in some patients with a stenosis in small vessels with little downstream myocardium at risk, complete revascularization may not be necessary [1].

Recent studies have confirmed that an incomplete revascularization results in higher MACCE rates [10] and a lower rate of survival [11]. The outcome of patients with FFR (fractional flow reserve)-based decision on bypass grafting was ambivalent. One study demonstrated that FFR-guided CABG was associated with a lower number of graft anastomoses and a lower rate of on-pump surgery compared with angiography-guided CABG. This did not result in a higher event rate during up to 36 months of follow-up and was associated with a lower rate of angina [12]. In another study in patients with multiple complex coronary artery stenoses, bypasses were grafted only to vessels with hemodynamically relevant stenoses. These patients were compared to patients with complete anatomical revascularization, and no clinical outcome differences were detected after 6 months. However, many non-revascularized coronary arteries with stenoses with non-pathological FFR values developed relevant stenoses with pathological FFR values within only 6 months [13], so that preventive revascularization may be considered. In the randomized multicentre FUTURE trial (FUnctional Testing Underlying coronary REvascularization; NCT01881555), complete FFR guidance to decide on CABG versus PCI versus medical treatment in patients with complex multivessel disease should be evaluated. In comparison to the angiography-guided group, FFR-directed decision resulted in significantly increased 1-year-mortality so that the trial was discontinued. In this context, it is noteworthy that FFR guidance resulted in downgrading of the complexity of coronary disease in many patients so that the rate of decision for CABG was lower.

Complete anatomical revascularization seems to be advantageous, probably since it does not only result in acute elimination of ischemia by bypassing a current critical stenosis. In fact, the life-prolonging effect first of all may be caused by an effective protection against myocardial infarction, including infarction by newly developed stenoses [14, 15]. Based on this idea, the term "surgical collaterals" was recently created [14]. A coronary bypass is commonly anastomosed to the periphery of a coronary artery and ensures peripheral myocardial perfusion even in case of proximal coronary plaque rupture and occlusion. In conclusion, the more plaques can be found in the coronary arteries (patients with a high Syntax score, particularly in diabetes mellitus), the more patients will profit from complete revascularization in general [16] and especially by means of CABG [14], whereat arterial revascularization is of particular importance [17]. Taken together, independently of the surgical approach—minimally invasive, off-pump or on-pump—a complete anatomical revascularization should be achieved.

Essentials:
- Complete revascularization should be pursued, especially in case of complex coronary pathology and patients with diabetes mellitus.
- The extent of surgical revascularization in patients with a high operation risk (e.g. with high STS score) may be reduced towards an incomplete revascularization (e.g. MIDCAB) or to a hybrid concept of MICS and additional PCI (e.g. hybrid MIDCAB) to minimize the operation risk.

## 2.2   Bypass Material

Another aspect of modern bypass surgery is arterial revascularization. Various studies [18, 19, 20] showed consistently that RA and BITA bypasses exhibit significantly lower mid- and long-term occlusion rates and consequently a higher patency rate compared to SV grafts, and thus, beneficially impact the clinical outcome. Therefore, a class I, level B recommendation is given for the left ITA (LITA) bypass to the LAD, and for the additional use of the RA instead of the SV in case of severe stenoses [1]. Extended arterial revascularization with the right ITA (RITA) has a class IIa, level B recommendation [1], whereas it is controversially discussed whether these arterial bypass constructions provide an improved long-term outcome compared to combined arterial and venous grafting. The use of a third arterial conduit in CABG patients is not associated with higher operative risk and is associated with superior long-term survival, irrespective of sex or diabetes mellitus [19]. Recently, the 10-years follow-up data of the ART study (Arterial Revascularization Trial) were published [21]. There were no significant differences regarding life expectancy between patients with BITA and a control group with only one ITA and additional other grafts, although it has to be mentioned that 20% of the control group had an RA graft as additional bypass. Unfortunately, there were further methodological limitations in this study so that the results of the currently recruiting multi-centre ROMA trial (Randomization Of single vs Multiple Arterial grafts; NCT03217006) will be of high interest. In a network meta-analysis, the use of SV was associated with a higher rate of adverse events after 5 years compared with RA [18]. In another study, the use of the RA or the RITA as second graft was associated with a similar and statistically significant long-term clinical benefit compared to the SV [22]. There were no differences in operative risk or complications between the two arterial conduits, but deep sternal wound infection remains a concern with BITA when skeletonization is not used. It has been reported that in case of OPCAB, SV have lower patency rates compared to arterial bypasses although the reasons remain unclear [23].

It was shown that dual anti-platelet therapy (DAPT) improves early mortality outcome and reduces SV graft failure without increasing early bleeding complications [24]. However, according to current guidelines, it is not yet generally recommended. Besides intrinsic biological resistance of the arteries against degenerative processes under arterial blood pressure, there may be a protective effect of arterial grafts on the coronary system, preventing progression of atherosclerosis in the native coronary vessels [25]. Sequential bypasses on several (up to five) and delicate coronary arteries with a calibre of approximately 1 mm profit especially from arterial grafting with excellent long-term outcome [26]. Due to higher resistance of vein grafts towards competitive flow, in case of complete revascularization and therewith the necessity of revascularization of territories with coronary arteries with a preserved native flow, vein grafts remain essential even in modern CABG.

Promising strategies follow the idea of modifying vein grafts to achieve improved adaption to the arterial blood pressure system and to reduce early atherosclerotic degeneration. With the implementation of the so-called no-touch vein harvesting technique, a patency rate of approximately 90% after 16 years could be achieved [27], so that this technique has received a class IIa, level B recommendation when open harvesting is used anyway [1]. With this approach, the perivascular tissue is preserved, which probably supports the integrity of the endothelial wall of the vein during arterialization. A negative aspect of the no-touch vein harvesting technique is the increased risk of wound infection due to the extended tissue defect and the impossibility of endoscopic vein harvesting (EVH), the latter of which has a general class IIa, level A recommendation to reduce the incidence of wound complications. Therefore, an individualized strategy is advisable: patients with very low wound infection risk (no trophic disorders or diabetes mellitus) and the necessity of a vein graft bypass may profit from a no-touch vein graft, whereas patients with risk factors for wound infection should receive EVH. Another option to protect vein grafts is an external stenting system that counteracts increased wall shear stress, a trigger of intima hyperplasia and atherosclerotic degeneration after arterialization of the vein. First clinical studies on the performance of externally stented veins versus non-stented grafts have yielded positive results so that a CE marking (Conformité Européenne) could be obtained [28].

Essentials:
- Arterial revascularization with BITA and/or RA should be used particularly for younger patients.
- If a vein graft is required, for elderly patients and patients with risks factors for wound infections, EVH is essential, while otherwise, no-touch vein harvesting is an alternative.
- External vein stents may be used to avoid graft dilatation and degeneration.

## 2.3    Bypass Architecture

A disadvantage of arterial bypass grafts is the vulnerability for dysfunctions, which aggravates with increased competitive flow in the native coronary system [29]. Due to the pronounced muscle layer, especially the RA shows an increased risk of spasms and bypass occlusion in case of high resistance in the native coronary system. Aortocoronary SV to the right coronary artery (RCA) showed better patency rates compared to arterial grafts, if there was a relevant residual flow rate (minimal lumen diameter >0.5 mm) in the native RCA [30]. In a systematic review of postoperative angiographies, the following factors were mentioned to be relevant for bypass dysfunctions in Y-grafts: degree of native vessel stenosis (odds ratio [OR] 0.66 per 10% increase), anatomic territory grafted (left circumflex artery (CX) OR 2.64, RCA OR 6.73 versus LAD), and end-to-side free wall anastomoses (OR 1.98) predicted anastomotic occlusion [31]. The LAD graft patency was unaffected by sequential grafting. Thus, the outcome of BITA Y-grafting is similar to that for other BITA configurations. The rate of arterial graft dysfunction decreases over time. Although competitive flow affects anastomotic patency, there is no threshold at which the risk of occlusion substantially increases.

Regardless of these risk factors for bypass dysfunctions in case of composite grafts, a retrospective propensity score-based analysis demonstrated a similar outcome after 20 years comparing BITA as composite graft to *in situ* grafts [32].

Thus, the clinical outcome of BITA grafting seems to be independent of the surgical configuration.

Even in patients with indication for totally arterial revascularization, an additional vein graft may be considered under special conditions. Particularly when an RA or the RITA is used in a T- or Y-graft configuration, the risk of bypass dysfunction may be relevant due to high intrinsic resistance resulting from the total length of the graft. Thus, constructing sequential or composite arterial grafts to vessels with asymmetric competitive flow should be avoided. In this scenario, downstream-anastomosed coronary arteries may not be adequately perfused [33]. At least, the most peripheral anastomosis should connect to the coronary artery with the least competitive flow. This is the reason why for example in MV-MICS, an RA composite graft (instead of an aortic graft) is only reasonable in case of high grade stenosis in the CX or RCA.

With a composite graft originating from the LITA, the complete coronary artery perfusion can be guaranteed generating a single inflow constellation. Due to the capability of adaption of the LITA, conformable to experimental studies, sufficient flow is expected to develop [25], whereas it has been also reported that regional hypoperfusion may occur under cardiac stress [34]. Therefore, in young patients, a double or triple inflow configuration should be preferred. For planned arterial revascularization, an aortic no-touch versus an aortocoronary bypass approach can be discussed [35]. A proven double inflow concept is composed of a LITA bypass to the left coronary artery, optionally equipped with an RA composite graft, and RCA revascularization by an *in situ* RITA elongated with a segment of the RA [35].

Essentials:
- A BITA composite graft allows for CABG without any aortocoronary anastomosis in complex multivessel disease.
- In case of low degree stenosis and the risk of asymmetric/competitive flow, composite grafts and sequential grafts should be avoided.
- For young patients with high performance requirements, a multiple inflow constellation should be preferred.

- In patients with low grade atherosclerotic aortic disease, an aortocoronary vein or (for younger patients) artery graft can be an option.
- An elongation of the RITA with a segment of the RA enhances the diversity of technical options for *in situ* grafts.
- For revascularization of the RCA, an arterial graft or venous composite graft is only reasonable in case of a minimal residual flow (minimal lumen diameter <0.5 mm) or total or subtotal occlusion, respectively.

## 2.4   Operative Risk Reduction

### 2.4.1   OPCAB

OPCAB allows for avoidance of CPB, which potentially reduces extracorporeal circulation-associated complications, such as systemic inflammatory response syndrome, procoagulatory activation leading to thrombosis and peripheral embolism, local vessel damage or air embolism. While several observational studies demonstrate advantages of OPCAB, prospective randomized studies could not yet confirm clinical long-term benefits. Recently, the impact of surgical experience was clearly demonstrated in a meta-analysis [36]. Decisive for the outcome after OPCAB, which remarkably challenges surgeons and anaesthetists compared to on-pump surgery on a resting empty heart, is the expertise of the surgical team. One of many challenges in off-pump surgery is the construction of the anastomoses on the lateral and posterior wall. Insufficient technical abilities may lead to low quality anastomoses, already detectable by intraoperative flow measurements [37]. The training in OPCAB and MICS should be based on CME (continuing medical education) standards, which means that the training should include the transfer of surgical and anaesthesiological standards as well as the manual training of the surgeons, so that the quality of the bypass anastomoses, the completion of revascularization and the hemodynamic stability of the patients can be guaranteed in any case and at all times [36]. In an experienced team with excellent knowledge, almost every operation can be conducted without a heart lung machine while achieving constant quality of the bypasses [7]. In any case, the expertise in OPCAB in a surgical team should be sufficient enough before handling a patient with relevant aortic calcification (please see the chapter on anaortic OPCAB) or by MICS (please see the chapter on trauma minimization) [38, 39].

In this book, we emphasize the need to adopt adequate techniques for anastomoses generation during off-pump and MICS procedures. The off-pump techniques described in this book are mainly based on standard operating procedures of the Leuven OPCAB school, developed by Paul Sergeant [40, 41] (https://campus.meplis.com/cabg/de/de/course/opcab-technique).

## 2.4.2    Anaortic OPCAB to Prevent Stroke

Early postoperative strokes mainly occur due to intraoperative embolization of aortic atherosclerotic plaques [42]. Observational studies and meta-analyses have indicated that improved outcome can be achieved by applying specific 'clampless' CABG strategies, including OPCAB with partial clamping, OPCAB with a proximal anastomotic device or the aortic no-touch technique, according to each patient's characteristics [43]. Our own experience in more than 6000 patients confirms that a consequent avoidance of any manipulation on the aorta, a so-called anaortic OPCAB technique, reduces the incidence of operative strokes below 1:1000 [44]. Totally arterial revascularization with BITA can be conducted in aortic no-touch technique to revascularize all possible targets on the anterior, lateral and posterior walls, as far as the RITA is long enough [45]. Also, in minimally invasive techniques with a singular ITA bypass or additional RA T-graft, no manipulation of the aorta is necessary. Since, as already mentioned, not every patient profits from such composite configurations, there are conditions favouring aortocoronary grafts, as long as the aorta exhibits no plaques (please see the chapter on epiaortic ultrasound).

## 2.4.3    Clampless OPCAB and Epiaortic Ultrasound Navigation

An alternative to the aortic no-touch technique or tangential clamping of the aorta is the clampless OPCAB technique. Here, by means of an anastomotic device, an aortocoronary bypass can be sutured without clamping the aorta. Afore, the aorta should be examined by epiaortic ultrasound imaging to detect plaques to minimize the risk of atherosclerotic embolization. In case of a high-grade atherosclerosis of the aorta (grade 3–5), an aortic no-touch technique should be preferred. The epiaortic ultrasound can also be used to detect plaque-free areas to connect the bypass to the aorta. It was proven that an examination with epiaortic ultrasound can reduce operative neurological complications [46].

According to Davila-Roman et al., the extent of atheromatosis of the aorta is usually categorized as mild to complex [47]. In brief, a *normal aorta* is defined by no identifiable intimal thickening; *mild atherosclerosis* is defined as intimal thickening ≤3.0 mm without intimal irregularities; *moderate atherosclerosis* as intimal thickening >3.0 mm with diffuse irregularities or calcification, or both; and *severe atherosclerosis* as intimal thickening ≥5.0 mm in addition to one or more of the following: large protruding atheromatous debris or thrombus, extensive calcification or ulcerated plaques. In our clinic, we utilize the slightly modified classification published by Halkos et al. [48] (Table 2.1).

In case of low-degree atherosclerosis (grade 1 or 2), assessed by systematic ultrasound imaging of the aorta, manipulation or even CPB cannulation and clamping may be acceptable. In this cohort of patients, there will probably be no differences in neurological outcome when clamping the aorta completely or partially in on-pump approaches as compared to partially clamping or clampless OPCAB [48].

TABLE 2.1 Ultrasound grading of atherosclerotic aortic plaques

| Ultrasound grade of ascending aorta atherosclerosis | Severity (atheroma thickness) | Description |
|---|---|---|
| 1 | Normal | Intimal thickness < 2 mm |
| 2 | Mild | Mild (focal or diffuse) intimal thickening of 2-3 mm |
| 3 | Moderate | Atheroma 3-5 mm (no mobile/ulcerated components) |
| 4 | Severe | Atheroma >5 mm (no mobile/ulcerated components) |
| 5 | Complex | Grade 2,3 or 4 atheroma plus mobile or ulcerated components |

Classification according to Davila-Roman et al. [47] and Halkos et al. [48]

Essentials:

• OPCAB is clearly indicated…

  – in case of significant calcification of the aorta. Clampless OPCAB or better anaortic OPCAB is essential, particularly to reduce the incidence of stroke.
  – in case of MICS, which means MIDCAB or MV-MICS

• Epiaortic ultrasound imaging is a powerful non-invasive tool to detect the local pattern of aortic plaques, which is a precondition for planning a safe operation strategy for an individual patient.
• Good expertise in OPCAB is essential for the whole surgical team.

## 2.5    Trauma Minimization

In order to minimize the surgical trauma, MICS approaches consisting of OPCAB procedures through mini-thoracotomies have been established, including hybrid solutions with MICS and additional PCI. Advantages particularly result from the avoidance of sternotomy, leading to enhanced thoracic stability and reduced wound size as well as wound infection risk.

*Left Anterolateral MIDCAB*

Single revascularization of the LAD with the LITA is the classical MIDCAB operation in case of a single-vessel coronary artery disease or a multivessel disease to be treated by hybrid techniques.

In *hybrid procedures*, stenoses of the CX or RCA are stented before or after a MIDCAB procedure. This method is practicable for multivessel disease patients with a high operative risk and CX/RCA stenoses eligible for PCI [1, 49].

To what extent a hybrid technique is an appropriate alternative to a complete anatomical revascularization by CABG in complex multivessel disease, is still unknown. Probably, it depends on the complexity of the coronary pathology and concomitant diseases, such as diabetes mellitus or ischemic cardiomyopathy [50]. In a small propensity-matched analysis comparing the 30-days-MACCE rates after hybrid versus complete surgical revascularization, no differences were found between both strategies [51]. In another study, 200 patients with multivessel coronary disease referred to conventional surgical revascularization were randomly assigned to undergo isolated CABG or a hybrid strategy. The primary endpoint was the occurrence of all-cause mortality within 5 years. Here, the hybrid group presented similar 5-year all-cause mortality when compared to conventional CABG [52]. A systematic review and meta-analysis of the studies comparing MIDCAB grafting with drug-eluting stent implantation in patients with isolated LAD disease showed that MIDCAB offers superior freedom from target vessel revascularization with similar mortality, myocardial infarction rate and MACCE compared to PCI [53]. The chronological order of PCI and CABG is an individual decision. PCI before a MIDCAB procedure provides the advantage of a reduced risk for intraoperative ischemia. On the other hand, the stent-associated preoperative DAPT is a problem. Depending on the interval between PCI and MIDCAB, a change or termination of the DAPT before the operation is advisable to avoid unnecessary bleeding complications and blood loss (Table 2.2). A respective delay of MIDCAB after PCI should be considered.

In case of non-critical stenoses and stable coronary situation in the CX and RCA, it is advisable to primarily conduct the MIDCAB procedure followed by PCI. Moreover, the result of the MIDCAB procedure can be controlled afterwards with angiography.

*Right Anterolateral MIDCAB*

A single revascularization of the RCA is possible. Due to calcification usually reaching until the distal part of the RCA, the usage of the RITA is possible only in a few cases. Otherwise, an aortocoronary bypass or a RITA elongation is recommended.

*MV-MICS*

This approach provides the possibility of complete anatomical revascularization in multivessel disease via a minimally invasive access. Although numerous MV-MICS studies have been published over the last 10 years [54], and the computed tomography-evaluated graft patency was excellent [55], there is still low evidence on this technique. Early postoperative regeneration and rehabilitation of the patients are the main goals, and have been confirmed in several patients series [56, 57].

Most frequently, MV-MICS is conducted with LITA to LAD and an additional bypass to the lateral and/or posterior wall as a composite T- or Y-graft from the LITA. Due to a difficult access to the RITA, usually an RA bypass or a vein graft is chosen in this context. The bypass architecture with a vein graft as T- or Y-graft from the LITA was recently published in a randomized study and also resulted in excellent patency rates [58]. Particularly in case of a non-appropriate RA, a vein graft is a good alternative and can be combined

TABLE 2.2 Management of platelet inhibition in case of hybrid procedures

| Drug | Approach |
|------|----------|
| *PCI <4 weeks* | |
| DAPT | In general, do not pause (critical evaluation) |
| ASA | Last intake 1 day before operation |
| Clopidogrel | Last intake 1 day before operation (critical evaluation) |
| Ticagrelor | Switch to clopidogrel (or tirofiban) |
| Prasugrel | Switch to clopidogrel (or tirofiban) |
| | |
| *PCI >4 weeks and <12 months* | |
| ASA | Last intake 1 day before operation |
| Ticagrelor | Last intake 4 days before operation |
| Clopidogrel | Last intake 6 days before operation |
| Prasugrel | Last intake 8 days before operation |
| | |
| *PCI <4 or >4 weeks + indication for oral anticoagulation* | |
| Phenprocoumon | Last intake 8 days before operation, bridging with heparin when INR <2 |
| NOAC | GFR $\geq$50 → last intake 3 days before operation GFR <50 → last intake 4 days before operation |

*PCI* Percutaneous coronary intervention, *DAPT* Dual antiplatelet therapy, *ASA* Acetylsalicylic acid, *INR* International normalized ratio, NOAC New oral anticoagulants, GFR Glomerular filtration rate (ml/min)

with the no-touch vein harvesting technique as well as with EVH to complete the minimally invasive concept. As already mentioned in the section „bypass architecture", in some MICS cases, an aortocoronary bypass is advisable. This technique was published by Chan [59]. In our clinic, we use an anastomotic device instead of tangential clamping. Of course, it is essential that the aorta is free of plaques, so that a preoperative computed tomography diagnostic and/or an intraoperative epiaortic ultrasound imaging are obligatory.

The patient cohort for MV-MICS is different from that for classical left anterolateral MIDCAB. While classical MIDCAB procedures are feasible in almost every patient with corresponding coronary pathology, MV-MICS procedures require long coronary arteries with sufficient diameters in the periphery of the CX and RCA to anastomose them in their very distal part. Additionally, these patients should not have too many concomitant diseases, as the operation time and the complexity of the operation itself are already high. The left ventricular ejection fraction should be considerably >35%. Due to increasing experience in the field of MV-MICS procedures and our fan technique (please see the respective section in the techniques chapter) allowing for avoidance of single lung ventilation, the spectrum of patients is increasing [60]. Lately, also the usage of BITA via left anterolateral thoracotomy was propagated [61, 62]. However, since the technique of MV-MICS is established in only a few cardiosurgical centres, there is still low evidence on the postoperative outcome. Yet, it is probable that, due to the avoidance of sternotomy, the regeneration und rehabilitation of the patients is accelerated. Therefore, and due to increasing patient demand, these techniques need to be further developed and evaluated [63].

Essentials:
- In principle, MIDCAB is possible in all patients with a single vessel coronary disease affecting the LAD.
- MIDCAB as a hybrid solution can be conducted in patients with high operative risk or at patients' request for MICS and a coronary pathology eligible for additional PCI.
- In MICS, an additional bypass to a diagonal branch is usually possible without much effort.
- Right-sided MIDCAB procedures allow for revascularization of the RCA and its periphery, whereas in these cases, a vein graft can be used instead of the RITA due to the mostly insufficient length of the RITA. Alternatively, the RITA bypass can be prolonged by an end-to-end anastomosis with a segment of the RA.

- For revascularization of the CX or posterior descending artery (PDA) in MV-MICS, either a central anastomosis to the aorta or a composite graft can be used, dependent predominantly on the degree of competitive flow.
- MV-MICS presupposes an appropriate anatomy of the coronary arteries and, due to the already high complexity of the procedure, low operative risk. Furthermore, the patients' request for MICS has become an important argument.

# References

1. Neumann FJ, Sousa-Uva M, Ahlsson A, et al. 2018 ESC/EACTS guidelines on myocardial revascularization. Eur Heart J. 2019;40:87–165.
2. Filardo G, Hamman BL, Da Graca B, et al. Efficacy and effectiveness of on- versus off-pump coronary artery bypass grafting: a meta-analysis of mortality and survival. J Thorac Cardiovasc Surg. 2018;155(1):172–9.
3. Takagi H, Ando T, Mitta S, et al. Meta-analysis comparing ≥10-year mortality of off-pump versus on-pump coronary artery bypass grafting. Am J Cardiol. 2017;120:1933–8.
4. Gaudino M, Benedetto U, Bakaeen F, et al. Off-versus on-pump coronary surgery and the effect of follow-up length and surgeons' experience: a meta-analysis. J Am Heart Assoc. 2018;7:e010034.
5. Benedetto U, Lau C, Caputo M, et al. Comparison of outcomes for off-pump versus on-pump coronary artery bypass grafting in low-volume and high-volume centers and by low-volume and high-volume surgeons. Am J Cardiol. 2018;121:552–7.
6. Chikwe J, Lee T, Itagaki S, et al. Long-term outcomes after off-pump versus on-pump coronary artery bypass grafting by experienced surgeons. J Am Coll Cardiol. 2018;72:1478–86.
7. Puskas JD, Williams WH, Mahoney EM, et al. Off-pump vs conventional coronary artery bypass grafting: early and 1-year graft patency, cost, and quality-of-life outcomes: a randomized trial. JAMA. 2004;291:1841–9.
8. Jones EL, Weintraub WS. The importance of completeness of revascularization during long-term follow-up after coronary artery operations. J Thorac Cardiovasc Surg. 1996;112:227–37.
9. Garcia S, Sandoval Y, Roukoz H, et al. Outcomes after complete versus incomplete revascularization of patients with multives-

sel coronary artery disease: a meta-analysis of 89,883 patients enrolled in randomized clinical trials and observational studies. J Am Coll Cardiol. 2013;62:1421–31.

10. Lee Y, Ohno T, Uemura Y, et al. Impact of complete revascularization on long-term outcomes after coronary artery bypass grafting in patients with left ventricular dysfunction. Circ J. 2018;83:122–9.

11. Diegeler A, Borgermann J, Kappert U, et al. Five-year outcome after off-pump or on-pump coronary artery bypass grafting in elderly patients. Circulation. 2019;139:1865–71.

12. Toth G, De Bruyne B, Casselman F, et al. Fractional flow reserve-guided versus angiography-guided coronary artery bypass graft surgery. Circulation. 2013;128:1405–11.

13. Thuesen AL, Riber LP, Veien KT, et al. Fractional flow reserve versus angiographically-guided coronary artery bypass grafting. J Am Coll Cardiol. 2018;72:2732–43.

14. Doenst T, Haverich A, Serruys P, et al. PCI and CABG for treating stable coronary artery disease: JACC review topic of the week. J Am Coll Cardiol. 2019;73:964–76.

15. Velazquez EJ, Lee KL, Jones RH, et al. Coronary-artery bypass surgery in patients with ischemic cardiomyopathy. N Engl J Med. 2016;374:1511–20.

16. Zimarino M, Ricci F, Romanello M, et al. Complete myocardial revascularization confers a larger clinical benefit when performed with state-of-the-art techniques in high-risk patients with multivessel coronary artery disease: a meta-analysis of randomized and observational studies. Catheter Cardiovasc Interv. 2016;87:3–12.

17. Raza S, Sabik JF 3rd, Masabni K, et al. Surgical revascularization techniques that minimize surgical risk and maximize late survival after coronary artery bypass grafting in patients with diabetes mellitus. J Thorac Cardiovasc Surg. 2014;148:1257–64; discussion 1264-1256.

18. Gaudino M, Benedetto U, Fremes S, et al. Radial-artery or saphenous-vein grafts in coronary-artery bypass surgery. N Engl J Med. 2018;378:2069–77.

19. Gaudino M, Puskas JD, Di Franco A, et al. Three arterial grafts improve late survival: a meta-analysis of propensity-matched studies. Circulation. 2017;135:1036–44.

20. Benedetto U, Raja SG, Albanese A, et al. Searching for the second best graft for coronary artery bypass surgery: a network

meta-analysis of randomized controlled trialsdagger. Eur J Cardiothorac Surg. 2015;47:59–65; discussion 65

21. Taggart DP, Benedetto U, Gerry S, et al. Bilateral versus single internal-thoracic-artery grafts at 10 years. N Engl J Med. 2019;380:437–46.

22. Gaudino M, Lorusso R, Rahouma M, et al. Radial artery versus right internal thoracic artery versus saphenous vein as the second conduit for coronary artery bypass surgery: a network meta-analysis of clinical outcomes. J Am Heart Assoc. 2019;8:e010839.

23. Zhang B, Zhou J, Li H, et al. Comparison of graft patency between off-pump and on-pump coronary artery bypass grafting: an updated meta-analysis. Ann Thorac Surg. 2014;97:1335–41.

24. Deo SV, Dunlay SM, Park SJ. Dual antiplatelet therapy after coronary artery bypass grafting: does off/on-pump play a role? Am J Cardiol. 2014;113:1085.

25. Dimitrova KR, Hoffman DM, Geller CM, et al. Arterial grafts protect the native coronary vessels from atherosclerotic disease progression. Ann Thorac Surg. 2012;94:475–81.

26. Nakajima H, Kobayashi J, Toda K, et al. Safety and efficacy of sequential and composite arterial grafting to more than five coronary branches in off-pump coronary revascularisation: assessment of intra-operative and angiographic bypass flow. Eur J Cardiothorac Surg. 2010;37:94–9.

27. Samano N, Geijer H, Liden M, et al. The no-touch saphenous vein for coronary artery bypass grafting maintains a patency, after 16 years, comparable to the left internal thoracic artery: a randomized trial. J Thorac Cardiovasc Surg. 2015;150:880–8.

28. Taggart DP, Webb CM, Desouza A, et al. Long-term performance of an external stent for saphenous vein grafts: the VEST IV trial. J Cardiothorac Surg. 2018;13:117.

29. Glineur D, Hanet C. Competitive flow and arterial graft a word of caution. Eur J Cardiothorac Surg. 2012;41:768–9.

30. Glineur D, D'hoore W, De Kerchove L, et al. Angiographic predictors of 3-year patency of bypass grafts implanted on the right coronary artery system: a prospective randomized comparison of gastroepiploic artery, saphenous vein, and right internal thoracic artery grafts. J Thorac Cardiovasc Surg. 2011;142:980–8.

31. Robinson BM, Paterson HS, Naidoo R, et al. Bilateral internal thoracic artery composite Y grafts: analysis of 464 angiograms in 296 patients. Ann Thorac Surg. 2016;101:974–80.

32. Di Mauro M, Iaco AL, Allam A, et al. Bilateral internal mammary artery grafting: in situ versus Y-graft. Similar 20-year outcome. Eur J Cardiothorac Surg. 2016;50:729–34.
33. Nakajima H, Kobayashi J, Toda K, et al. A 10-year angiographic follow-up of competitive flow in sequential and composite arterial grafts. Eur J Cardiothorac Surg. 2011;40:399–404.
34. Sakaguchi G, Tadamura E, Ohnaka M, et al. Composite arterial Y graft has less coronary flow reserve than independent grafts. Ann Thorac Surg. 2002;74:493–6.
35. Buxton BF, Hayward PA. The art of arterial revascularization-total arterial revascularization in patients with triple vessel coronary artery disease. Ann Cardiothorac Surg. 2013;2:543–51.
36. Puskas JD, Gaudino M, Taggart DP. Experience is crucial in off-pump coronary artery bypass grafting. Circulation. 2019;139:1872–5.
37. Hassanein W, Albert AA, Arnrich B, et al. Intraoperative transit time flow measurement: off-pump versus on-pump coronary artery bypass. Ann Thorac Surg. 2005;80:2155–61.
38. Albert A, Sergeant P, Florath I, et al. Process review of a departmental change from conventional coronary artery bypass grafting to totally arterial coronary artery bypass and its effects on the incidence and severity of postoperative stroke. Heart Surg Forum. 2011;14:E73–80.
39. Sergeant P, Wouters P, Meyns B, et al. OPCAB versus early mortality and morbidity: an issue between clinical relevance and statistical significance. Eur J Cardiothorac Surg. 2004;25:779–85.
40. De Raet JM, Desimone JP, Sergeant PT. Off-pump coronary artery bypass grafting: anno 2011. Multimed Man Cardiothorac Surg. 2011;2011:713.
41. Desimone J, Sergeant P. Off-pump myocardial revascularization. Multimed Man Cardiothorac Surg. 2006;2006. https://doi.org/10.1510/mmcts.2004.000539.
42. Albert A, Peck EA, Wouters P, et al. Performance analysis of interactive multimodal CME retraining on attitude toward and application of OPCAB. J Thorac Cardiovasc Surg. 2006;131:154–62.
43. Kawajiri H, Yaku H, Glineur D, et al. Clampless versus clamped coronary bypass grafting: does it make a difference? Curr Opin Cardiol. 2017;32:737–43.
44. Albert A, Ennker J, Hegazy Y, et al. Implementation of the aortic no-touch technique to reduce stroke after off-pump coronary surgery. J Thorac Cardiovasc Surg. 2018;156(2):544–54.

45. Albert A, Hassanein W, Florath I, et al. Technical aspects of composite arterial T-grafts: estimation of required conduit length by a simple formula. Thorac Cardiovasc Surg. 2008;56:461–6.
46. Ikram A, Mohiuddin H, Zia A, et al. Does epiaortic ultrasound screening reduce perioperative stroke in patients undergoing coronary surgery? A topical review. J Clin Neurosci. 2018;50:30–4.
47. Davila-Roman VG, Murphy SF, Nickerson NJ, et al. Atherosclerosis of the ascending aorta is an independent predictor of long-term neurologic events and mortality. J Am Coll Cardiol. 1999;33:1308–16.
48. Halkos ME, Anderson A, Binongo JNG, et al. Operative strategies to reduce cerebral embolic events during on- and off-pump coronary artery bypass surgery: a stratified, prospective randomized trial. J Thorac Cardiovasc Surg. 2017;154(4):1278–85.
49. Fihn SD, Gardin JM, Abrams J, et al. 2012 ACCF/AHA/ACP/AATS/PCNA/SCAI/STS guideline for the diagnosis and management of patients with stable ischemic heart disease: executive summary: a report of the American College of Cardiology Foundation/American Heart Association task force on practice guidelines, and the American College of Physicians, American Association for Thoracic Surgery, Preventive Cardiovascular Nurses Association, Society for Cardiovascular Angiography and Interventions, and Society of Thoracic Surgeons. Circulation. 2012;126:3097–137.
50. Leviner DB, Torregrossa G, Puskas JD. Incomplete revascularization: what the surgeon needs to know. Ann Cardiothorac Surg. 2018;7:463–9.
51. Rosenblum JM, Harskamp RE, Hoedemaker N, et al. Hybrid coronary revascularization versus coronary artery bypass surgery with bilateral or single internal mammary artery grafts. J Thorac Cardiovasc Surg. 2016;151:1081–9.
52. Tajstra M, Hrapkowicz T, Hawranek M, et al. Hybrid coronary revascularization in selected patients with multivessel disease: 5-year clinical outcomes of the prospective randomized pilot study. JACC Cardiovasc Interv. 2018;11:847–52.
53. Raja SG, Uzzaman M, Garg S, et al. Comparison of minimally invasive direct coronary artery bypass and drug-eluting stents for management of isolated left anterior descending artery disease: a systematic review and meta-analysis of 7,710 patients. Ann Cardiothorac Surg. 2018;7:567–76.

54. Mcginn JT Jr, Usman S, Lapierre H, et al. Minimally invasive coronary artery bypass grafting: dual-center experience in 450 consecutive patients. Circulation. 2009;120(11 Suppl):S78–84.
55. Ruel M, Shariff MA, Lapierre H, et al. Results of the minimally invasive coronary artery bypass grafting angiographic patency study. J Thorac Cardiovasc Surg. 2014;147:203–8.
56. Rabindranauth P, Burns JG, Vessey TT, et al. Minimally invasive coronary artery bypass grafting is associated with improved clinical outcomes. Innovations. 2014;9:421–6.
57. Lapierre H, Chan V, Sohmer B, et al. Minimally invasive coronary artery bypass grafting via a small thoracotomy versus off-pump: a case-matched study. Eur J Cardiothorac Surg. 2011;40:804–10.
58. Kim KB, Hwang HY, Hahn S, et al. A randomized comparison of the Saphenous Vein Versus Right Internal Thoracic Artery as a Y-Composite Graft (SAVE RITA) trial: one-year angiographic results and mid-term clinical outcomes. J Thorac Cardiovasc Surg. 2014;148:901–7; discussion 907-908.
59. Chan V, Lapierre H, Sohmer B, et al. Handsewn proximal anastomoses onto the ascending aorta through a small left thoracotomy during minimally invasive multivessel coronary artery bypass grafting: a stepwise approach to safety and reproducibility. Semin Thorac Cardiovasc Surg. 2012;24:79–83.
60. Sixt S, Aubin H, Kalb R, et al. Continuous procedural full-lung ventilation during minimally invasive coronary bypass grafting. Ann Thorac Surg. 2017;104:1994–2000.
61. Diab M, Farber G, Sponholz C, et al. Coronary artery bypass grafting using bilateral internal thoracic arteries through a left-sided minithoracotomy: a single-center starting experience. Thorac Cardiovasc Surg. 2018;67:437.
62. Kikuchi K, Chen X, Mori M, et al. Perioperative outcomes of off-pump minimally invasive coronary artery bypass grafting with bilateral internal thoracic arteries under direct visiondagger. Interact Cardiovasc Thorac Surg. 2017;24:696–701.
63. Gaudino M, Bakaeen F, Davierwala P, et al. New strategies for surgical myocardial revascularization. Circulation. 2018;138:2160–8.

# Chapter 3
## Operative Techniques

**A. Albert, A. Assmann, and A. K. Assmann**

## 3.1 Graft Harvesting

### 3.1.1 Arterial Grafts

Left internal thoracic artery (LITA)
Right internal thoracic artery (RITA)
Radial artery (RA)
Right gastroepiploic artery (GEA)

A. Albert (✉)
Clinic of Dortmund gGmbH - Clinic for Heart Surgery,
Beurhausstraße, Germany
e-mail: alexander.albert@klinikumdo.de

A. Assmann · A. K. Assmann
Department of Cardiac Surgery, University Hospital Düsseldorf,
Düsseldorf, Nordrhein-Westfalen, Germany
e-mail: alexander.assmann@med.uni-duesseldorf.de; annakathrin.
assmann@med.uni-duesseldorf.de

© Springer Nature Switzerland AG 2021                                29
A. Albert et al. (eds.), *Operative Techniques in Coronary
Artery Bypass Surgery*,
https://doi.org/10.1007/978-3-030-48497-2_3

## 3.1.1.1   ITA Harvesting: Open

After entering the pleural space via a longitudinal incision of the mediastinal pleura, the parietal pleura is incised medially of the ITA while avoiding damage to the concomitant veins.

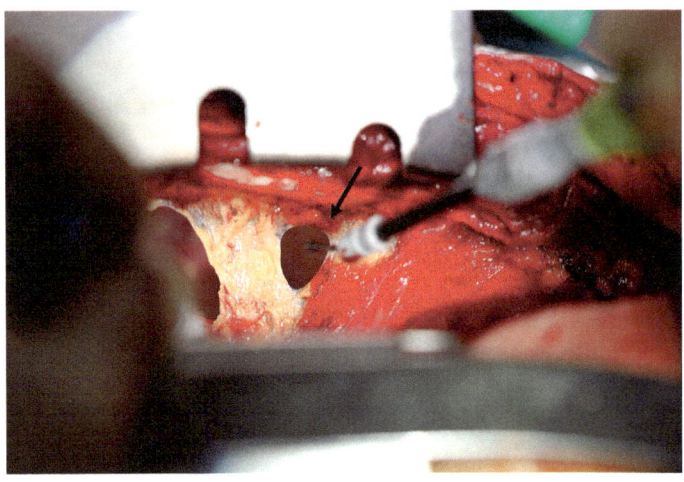

PHOTO 3.1: Mediastinal pleura incision
→, *pleura incision*

At the beginning of the preparation, the phrenic nerve should be exposed to keep adequate distance between the preparation zone and the nerve.

Using an electrocoagulation device tip or scissors, surrounding connective and adipose tissue as well as the internal thoracic veins are separated from the ITA following a skeletonization approach.

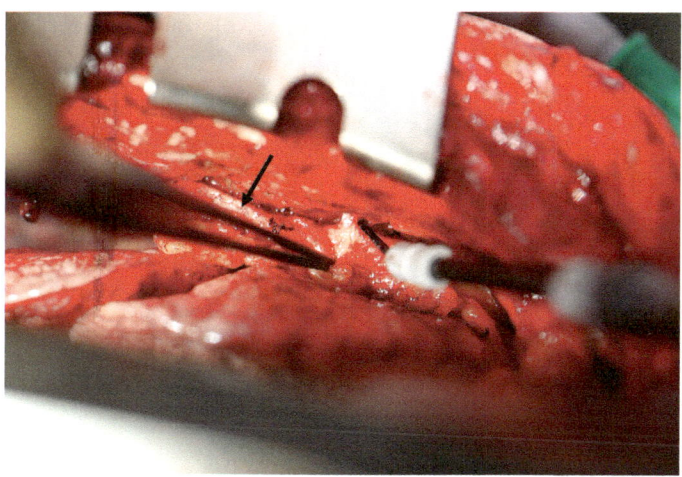

Photo 3.2: Tissue dissection
→, *ITA*

All branches are coagulated or closed by haemoclips paying attention to sufficient distance to the artery.

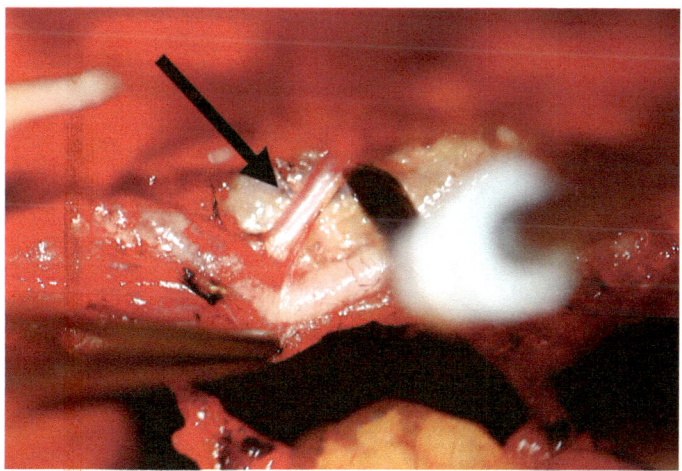

Photo 3.3: Branch coagulation
→, *side branch of the ITA*

After complete preparation, the skeletonized artery is tested for adequate blood flow.

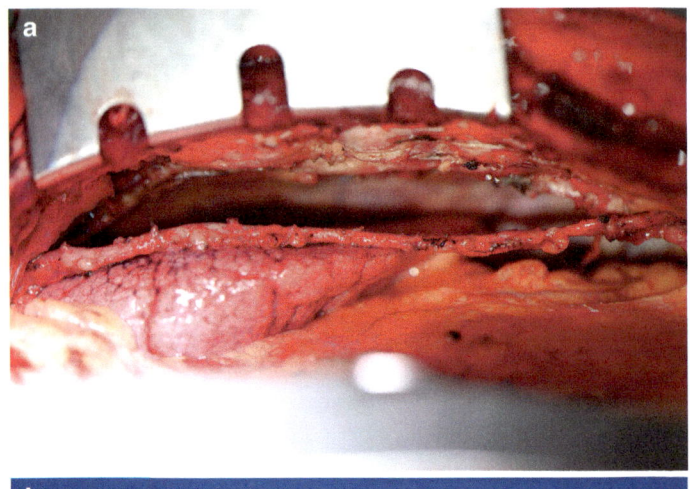

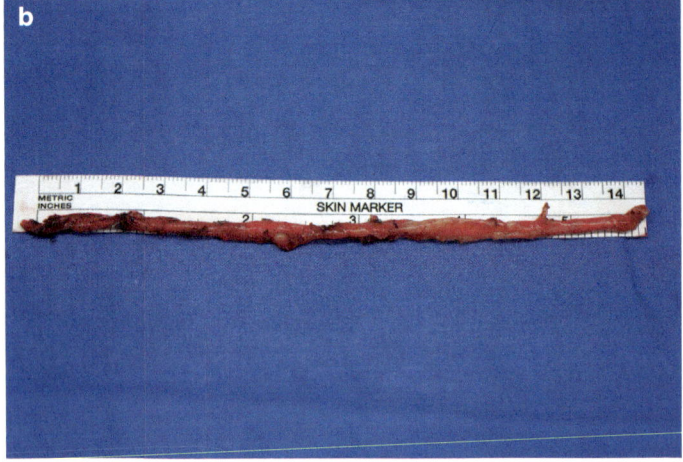

Photo 3.4a+b: Skeletonized ITA
*a: Skeletonized LITA in situ*
*b: Skeletonized RITA (free graft)*

## 3.1.1.2   RA Harvesting: Endoscopic

For endoscopic RA harvesting (ERAH), the following equipment is recommended.

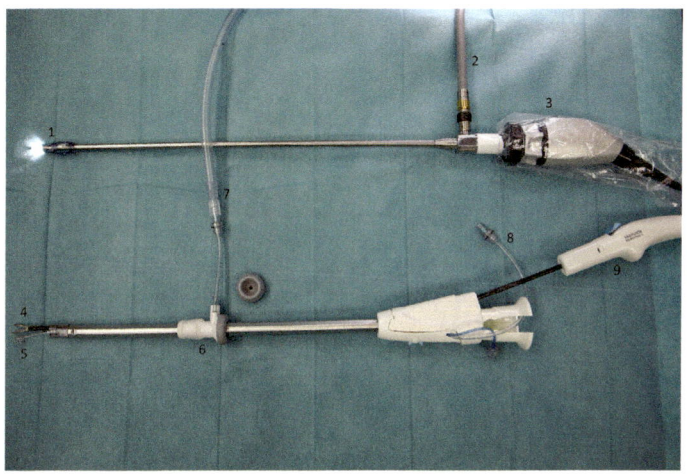

PHOTO 3.5:  Equipment
*1, conical dissection tip; 2, electric light cable; 3, endoscope camera; 4, thermostatic tip; 5, C-shaped bow; 6, port; 7 + 8, CO$_2$ insufflation connector; 9, handle* (Vasoview Hemopro 2, Getinge, Gothenburg, Sweden)

An incision (2–2.5 cm length) is made 1 cm proximally of the transverse carpal ligament in the longitudinal direction to get the access to the RA. The RA is separated from surrounding tissue as far as one can see through the incision. Whether the RA can be explanted without impairment of the hand perfusion, has to be checked before: The oxygen saturation pulse curve should not be flattened when the RA is clamped, indicating sufficient perfusion via the ulnar artery.

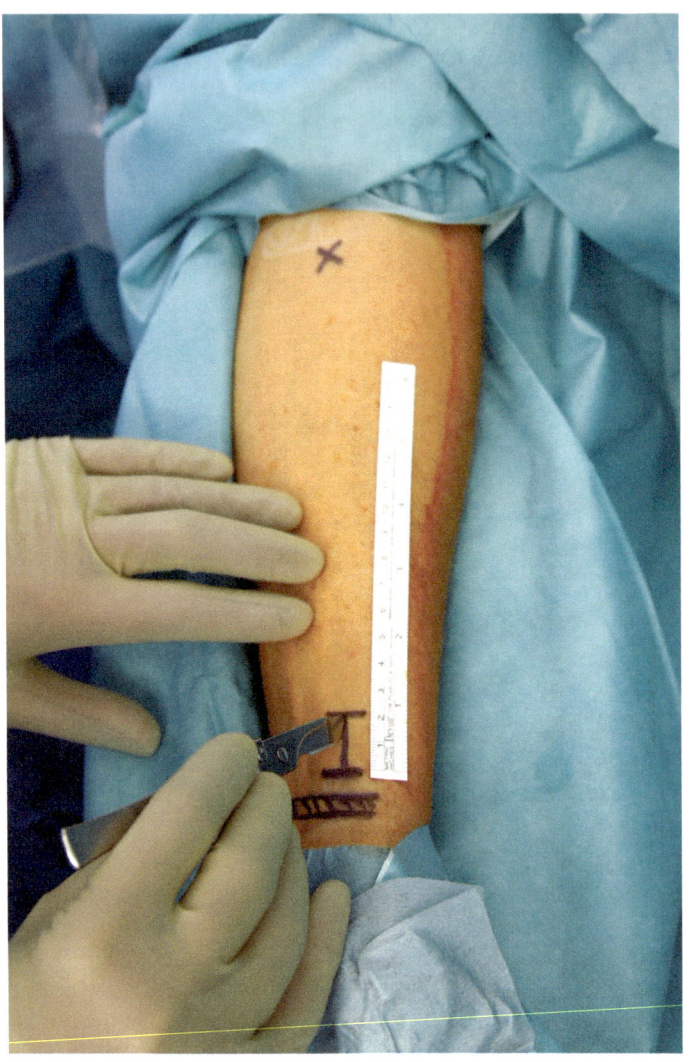

PHOTO 3.6:  Incision
*Incision proximally of the transverse carpal ligament*

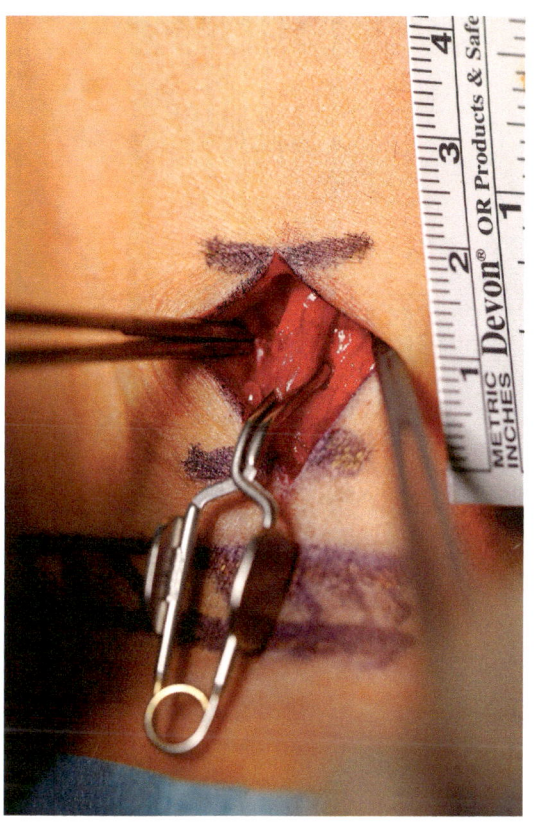

PHOTO 3.7: RA clamping
*RA clamping while monitoring the oxygen saturation pulse curve*

To start the preparation, the conical dissection tip together with the port is inserted through the small incision. Continuous $CO_2$ insufflation-mediated pressure in the preparation channel guarantees a good view by widening the generated tunnel.

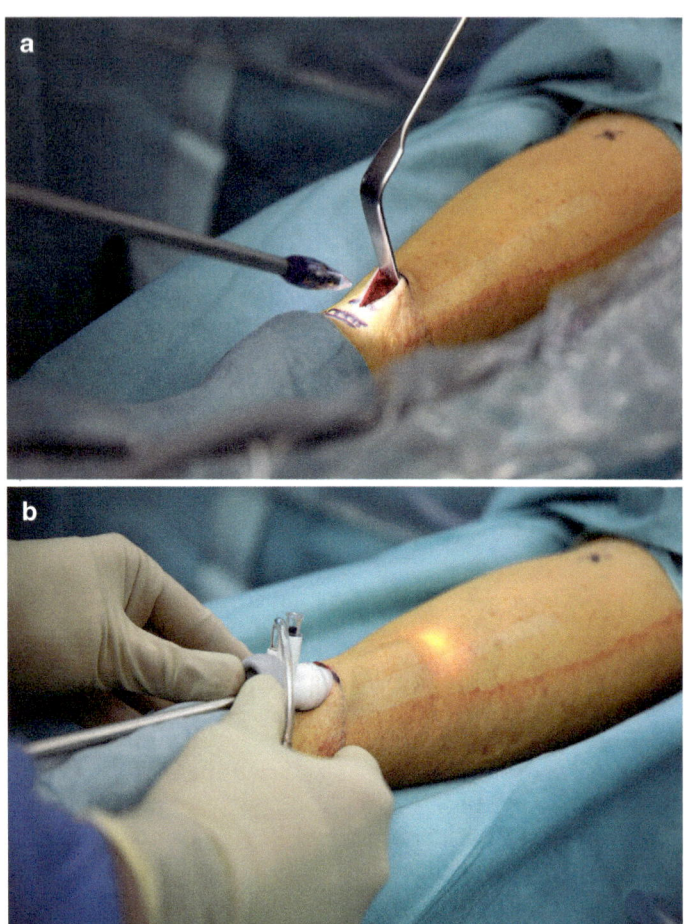

Photo 3.8a+b: Port insertion
*The conical dissection tip (a) together with the port (b) is inserted through the small incision*

Now the RA is separated thoroughly from the surrounding tissue on each side. All branches of the RA should be freed from connective and adipose tissue at least for a few millimetres so that they can be coagulated safely in the next step.

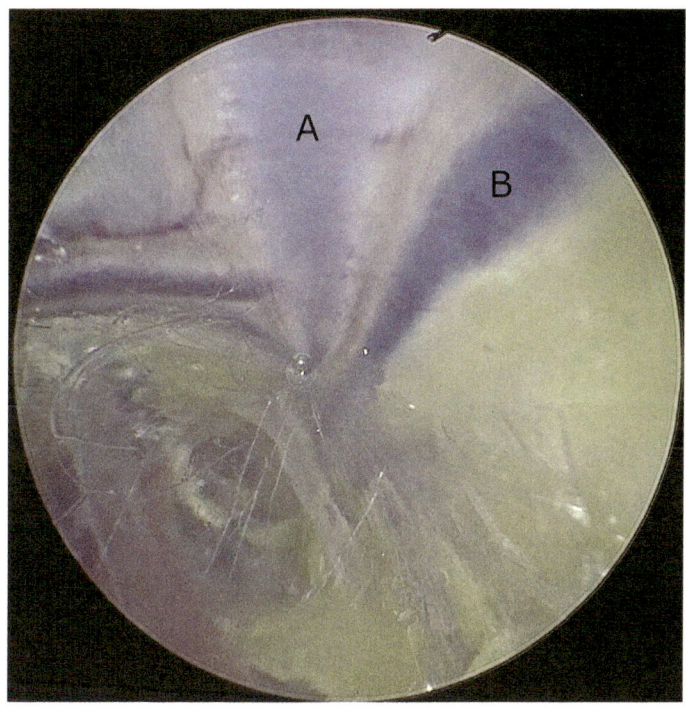

PHOTO 3.9: Tissue dissection
*Endoscopic view through the transparent conical dissection tip*
*A, RA; B, accompanying vein*

Before coagulation of the branches of the RA, a fasciotomy above the artery should be made to gain more space in
the tunnel for the endoscope.

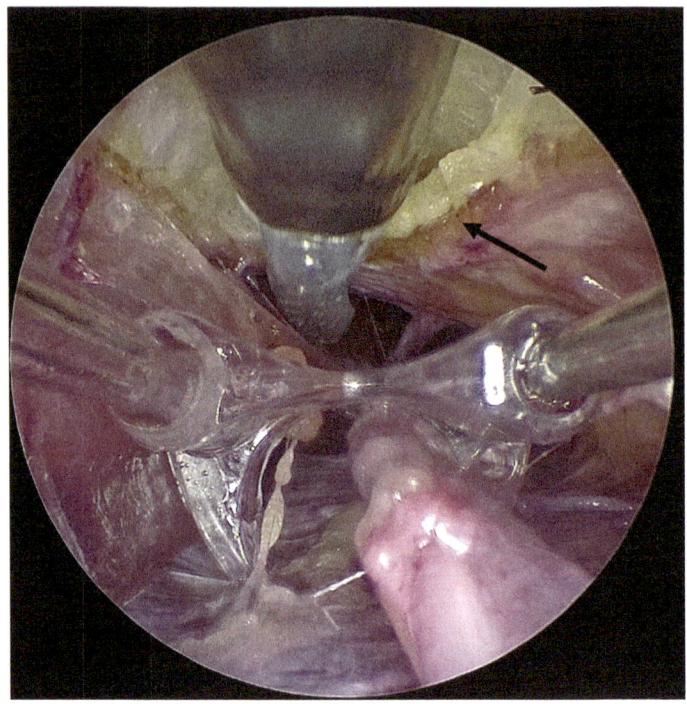

Photo 3.10: Fasciotomy to widen the tunnel
→, *fasciotomy*

Afterwards, all branches of the RA should be cut with the thermostatic tip. With a C-shaped bow, the RA is moved away when cutting a branch with the thermostatic tip so that the RA is not harmed.

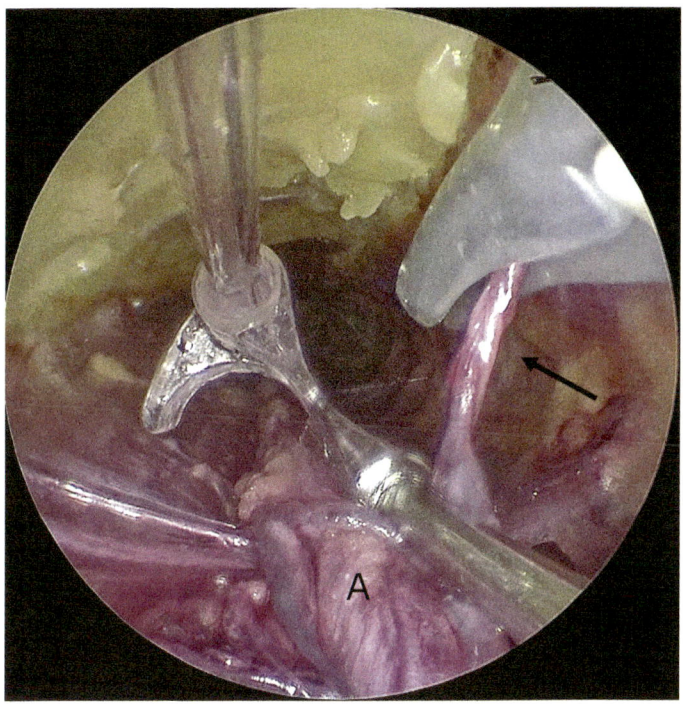

PHOTO 3.11: Branch coagulation
*A, RA; →, side branch*

When all branches are cut and the RA is completely separated from surrounding tissue, a little incision in the skin is
made at the end of the preparation channel. With a mosquito
clamp, the end of the RA is taken and then carefully pulled
out of the tunnel. On the distal side of the clamp, the RA is
cut so that the artery lapses into the tunnel again. The proximal end of the RA should be ligated sufficiently. The other
end of the prepared artery is caught with the C-bow and then
transported through the preparation tunnel towards the distal incision.

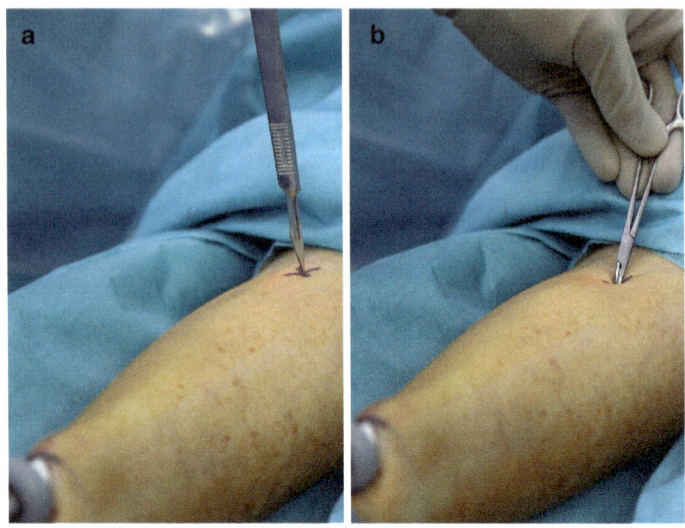

PHOTO 3.12A+B: Vessel extraction 1
*a: Incision at the end of the preparation channel*
*b: Mosquito clamp catches the RA*

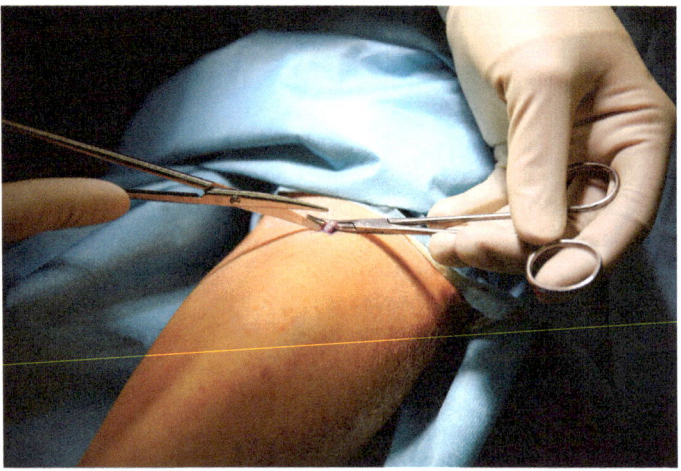

PHOTO 3.13: Vessel extraction 2 *RA is cut at the distal side of the clamp*

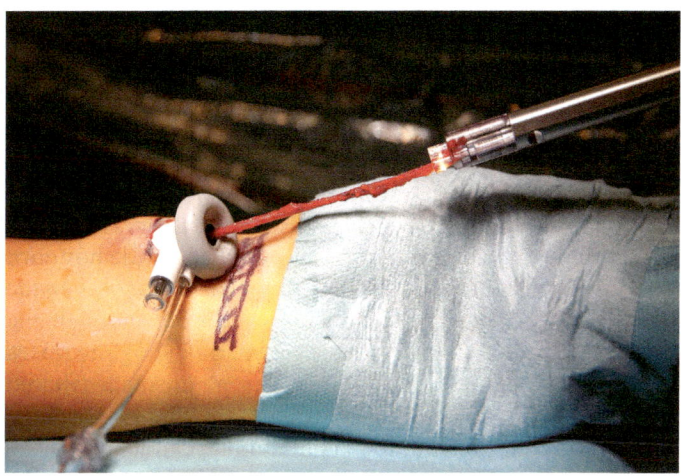

PHOTO 3.14: Vessel extraction 3
*Transportation of the RA out of the channel with the C-shaped bow*

Before closing the incision, a Redon drainage should be placed into the tunnel. Then, the incision is closed by sub- and intracutaneous sutures.

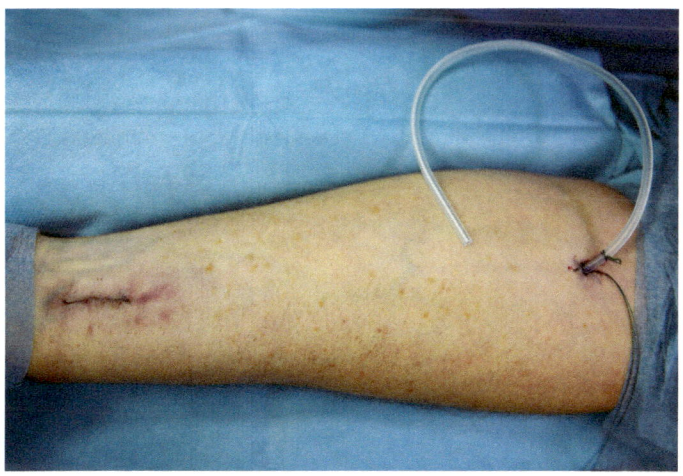

PHOTO 3.15: Cosmetic result
*Redon drainage is placed in the channel*

## 3.1.2   Vein Grafts

Great saphenous vein (GSV)
Small saphenous vein (SSV)

### 3.1.2.1   SV Harvesting: Open and No-Touch

If open vein harvesting (OVH) is chosen, a no-touch approach should be considered. A longitudinal skin incision is made directly above the GSV, leaving reasonable distance to the medial malleolus for lower risk of wound healing disorders. For the no-touch pedicle approach, the distance should exceed 5 cm to facilitate preservation of the saphenous nerve that in the distal lower limb is commonly attached to the GSV. In order to account for anatomical irregularities, the initial incision should not exceed a few centimetres.

After exposure of the GSV, a small pedicle is prepared using electrocoagulation or haemoclips. The saphenous nerve should be preserved. Following the course of the GSV, the skin is further incised and the pedicle explanted.

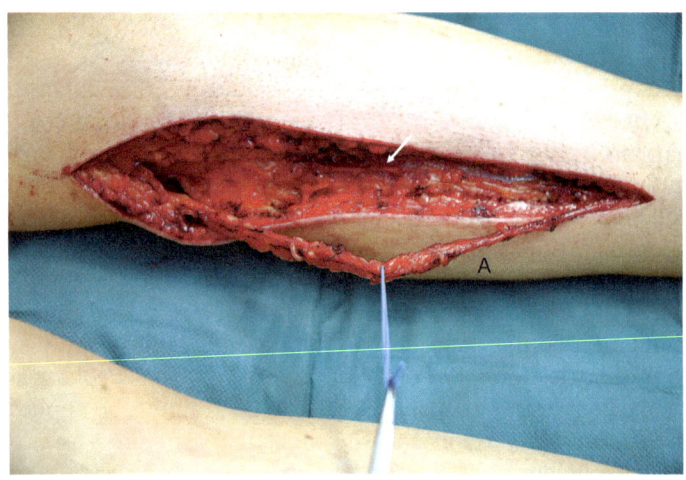

Photo 3.16:  Vein exposure
*A, GSV pedicle; →, saphenous nerve*

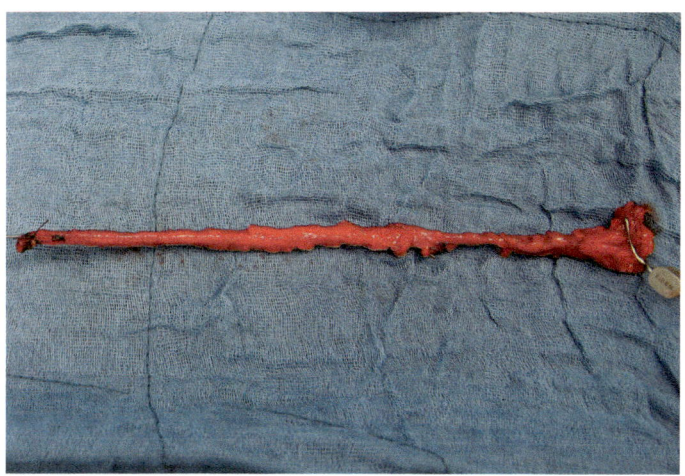

Photo 3.17: GSV pedicle

Before closing the incision, a Redon drainage may be considered depending on wound depth and bleeding status. Then, the incision is closed by sub- and intracutaneous sutures. Slight compression by sterile bandages is recommended at least for the intraoperative period of anticoagulation, whereas perfusion disorders, such as in peripheral arterial disease, have to be considered.

## 3.1.2.2   SV Harvesting: Endoscopic

For endoscopic vein harvesting (EVH), the above mentioned equipment is necessary as it should be used for ERAH. To start the preparation of the GSV, an incision of 2–2.5 cm in length is made below the medial tibial condyle. The SV is separated from surrounding tissue as far as one can see through the incision.

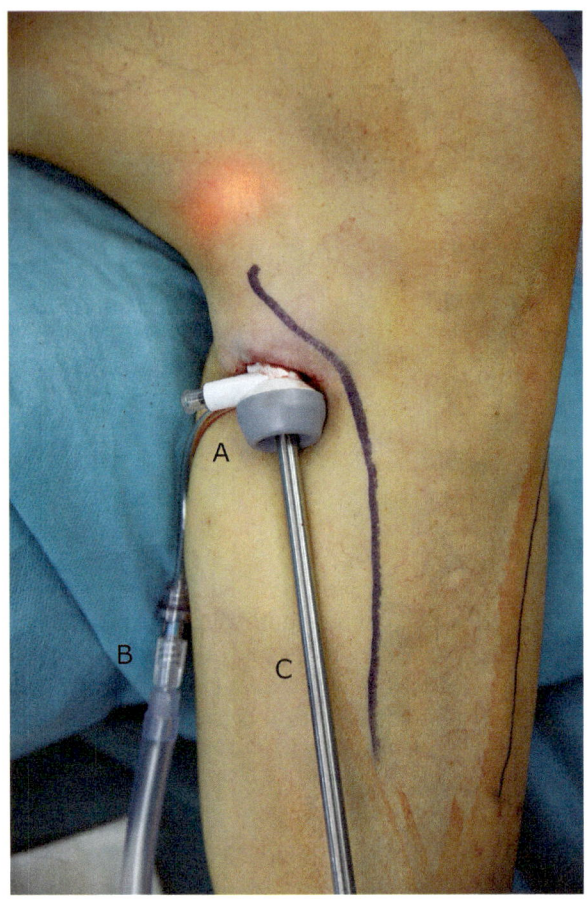

Photo 3.18: Access
*A, port; B, CO$_2$ insufflation; C, endoscope camera*

The conical dissection tip together with the port is inserted through the small incision. Continuous CO$_2$ insufflation-mediated pressure in the preparation channel guarantees a good view by widening the generated tunnel. Now the SV is separated thoroughly from the surrounding tissue on each side. All branches of the vein should be freed from connective and adipose tissue at least for a few millimetres so that they can be coagulated safely in the next step.

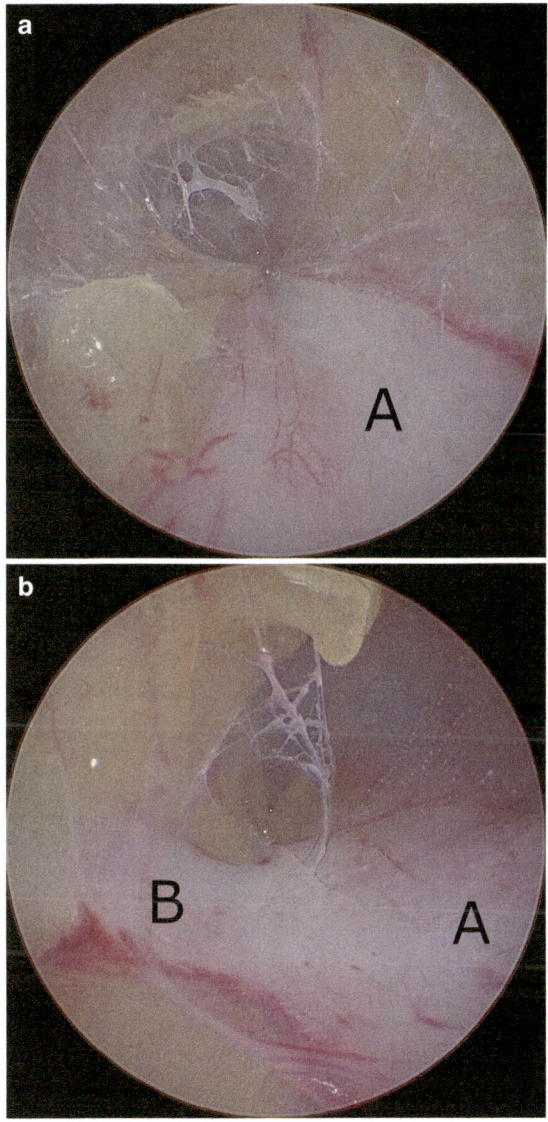

PHOTO 3.19A+B: Tissue dissection
*Endoscopic views through the transparent conical dissection tip*
*a: A, GSV*
*b: A, GSV; B, side branch of the GSV*

All branches of the GSV are coagulated by the thermostatic tip, while the GSV is carefully pushed away with the C-bow to minimize the risk of damage to the vein during this procedure.

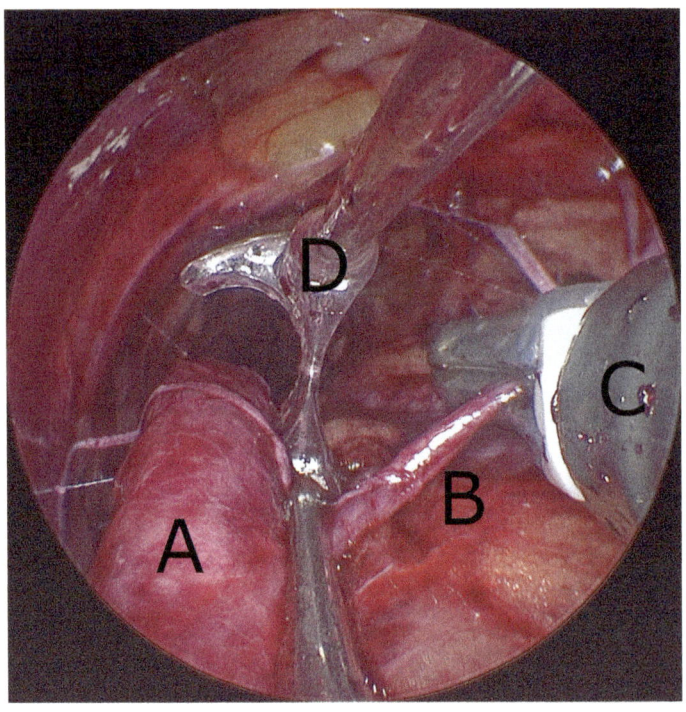

PHOTO 3.20: Branch coagulation
*A, GSV; B, side branch; C, thermostatic tip; D, C-shaped bow*

When all branches are cut and the GSV is completely separated from surrounding tissue, a little incision in the skin is made at the end of the preparation channel. With a mosquito clamp, the end of the SV is taken and then carefully pulled out of the tunnel. On the distal side of the clamp, the vein is cut so that it lapses into the tunnel again. The proximal end of the GSV should be ligated sufficiently. The other end of the prepared vessel is caught with the C-bow and then transported through the preparation tunnel towards the distal incision.

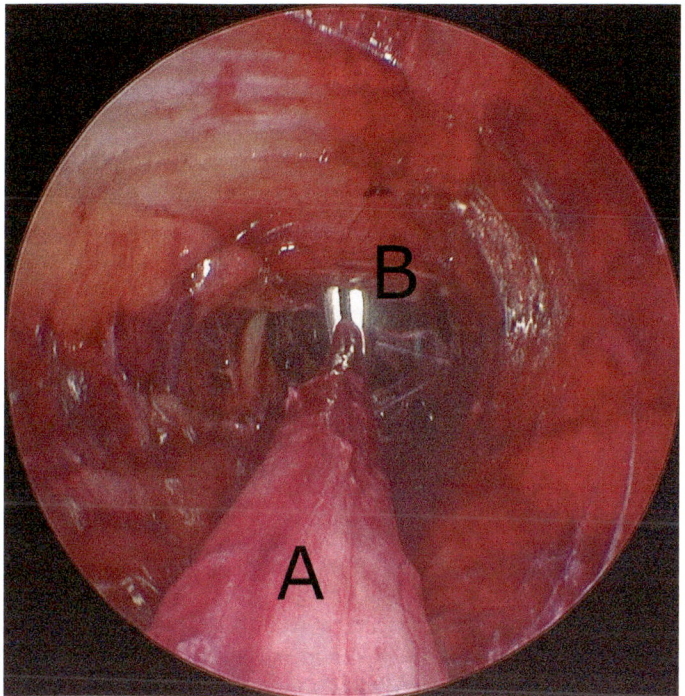

PHOTO 3.21: Vessel extraction
*A, GSV; B, mosquito clamp*

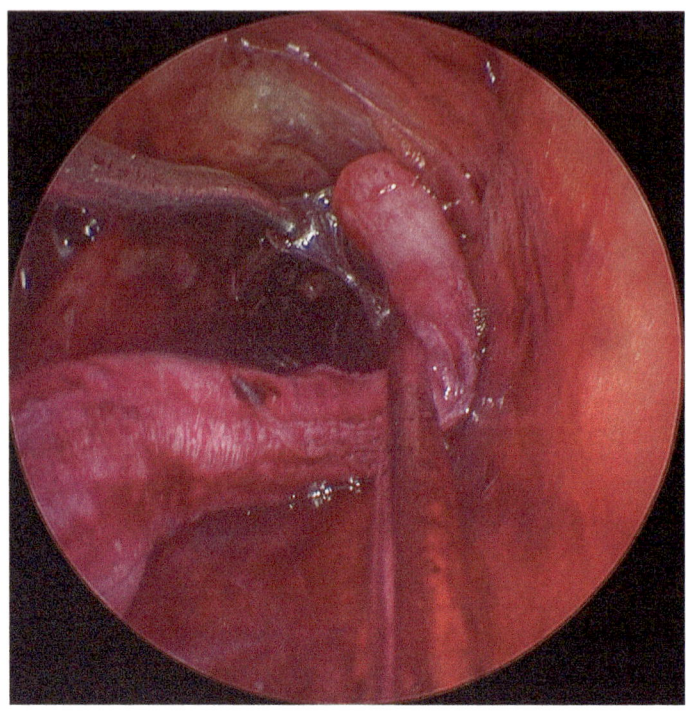

PHOTO 3.22: Vessel transportation
*Transportation of the GSV with the C-shaped bow*

Before closing the incision, a Redon drainage should be placed into the tunnel. Then, the incision is closed by sub- and intracutaneous sutures. Slight compression by sterile bandages is recommended at least for the intraoperative period of anticoagulation, whereas perfusion disorders, such as in peripheral arterial disease, have to be considered.

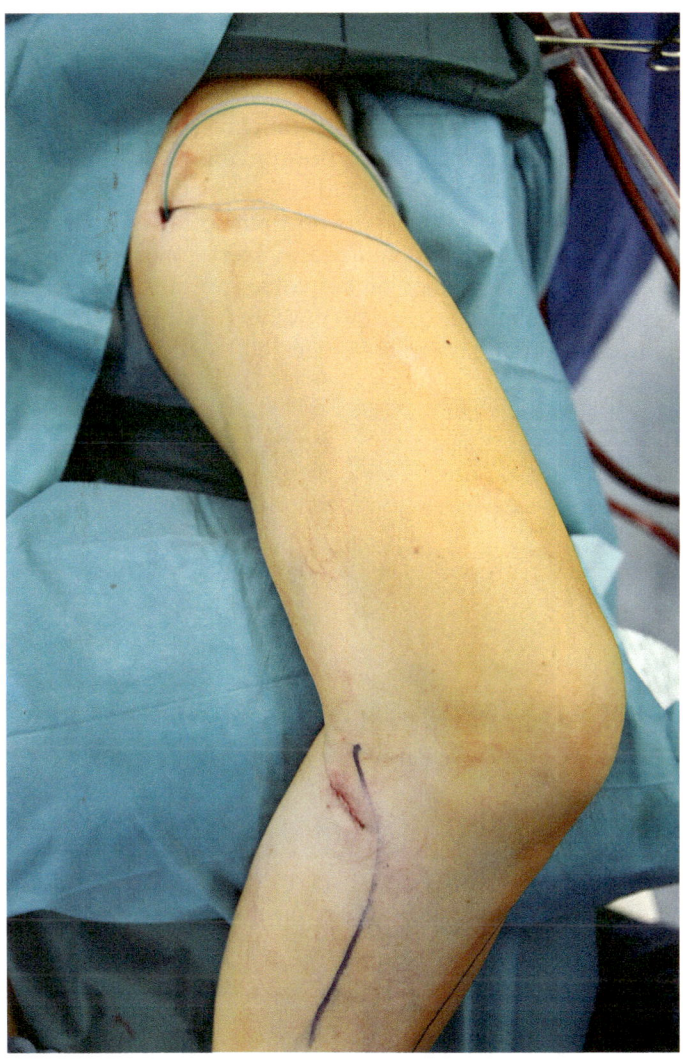

Photo 3.23: Cosmetic result

### 3.1.3  Further Graft Preparation

All grafts should be harvested and prepared very carefully considering that we are dealing with living tissue. For cannulation, the physiological blood flow direction has to be recapitulated, and the cannula should be equipped with a pressure control syringe in order not to apply unnecessarily high pressure to the graft. We recommend to exert a maximum pressure of 250 mmHg, since higher values are not expected to occur in the human circulation. Without pressure control, the applied pressure may easily exceed 1000 mmHg.

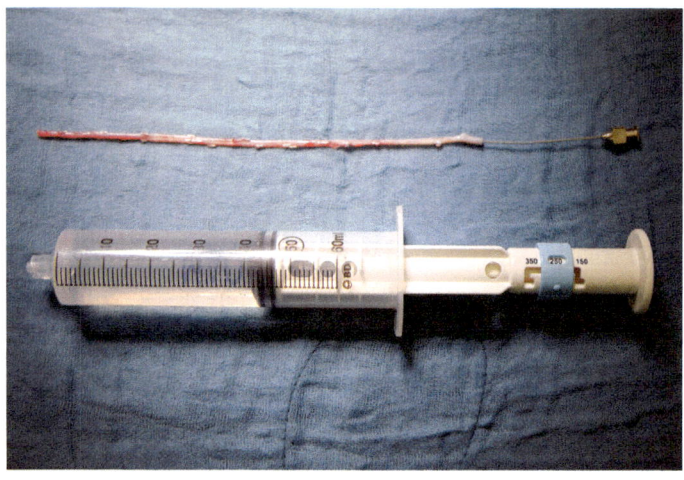

Photo 3.24: Pressure control syringe (Vasoshield, Getinge, Gothenburg, Sweden)

Local vasodilators such as papaverin may be administered into arterial grafts. All vessels should be stored in buffered solution with physiological pH value until implantation.

Preparation of the graft branches can be conducted by clipping or ligatures. In case of application of external stabilization devices (Photo 2), ligatures are required instead of clips. For vein graft anastomoses, vein valve-containing areas should be avoided.

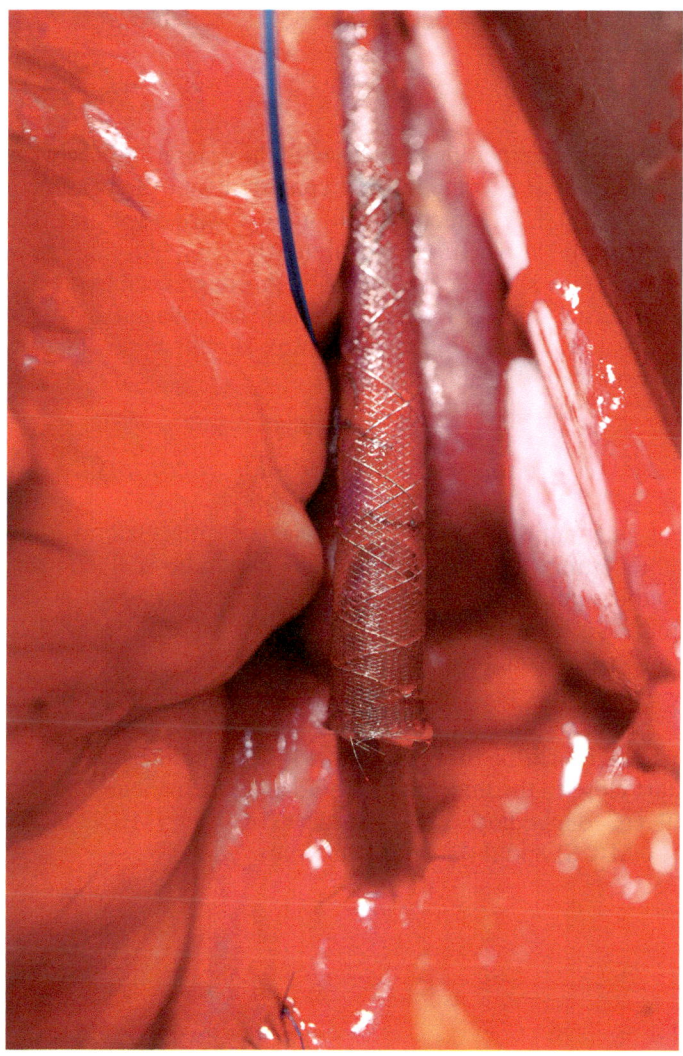

Photo 3.25: External stabilization device on a GSV graft (VEST, Vascular Graft Solutions, Tel Aviv, Israel)

## 3.2   Thoracic Access

### 3.2.1   Median Sternotomy

A median skin incision is made, with the cranial end as low as possible. After subcutaneous preparation, an exactly median sternotomy is conducted with utmost care regarding the retrosternal structures, particularly in redo surgery. Haemostasis should be achieved by thorough local treatment considering sternal haemostats, such as collagen matrices, whereas the utilization of bone wax should be avoided to prevent wound healing disorders.

### 3.2.2   Left Anterolateral Mini-Thoracotomy

For minimally invasive CABG via left anterolateral mini-thoracotomy, single lung ventilation should be enabled using double-lumen tubes or bronchus blockers. In case of inadequate gas exchange, double lung ventilation can be installed applying our fan technique described below.

Patients are placed in a supine position with the left thorax lifted up by 30°. A submammary skin incision is made following the fourth or fifth intercostal space. The incision should start close to the midclavicular line and reach a length of 5 to 10 cm, depending on the surgical method (MIDCAB or MV-MICS) and the patient's anatomy.

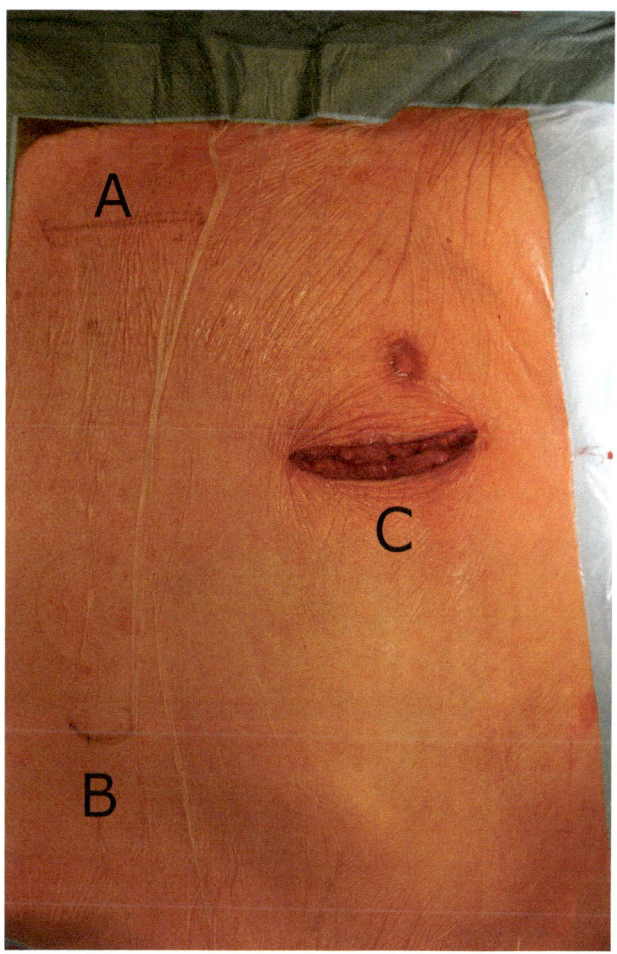

PHOTO 3.26: Skin incision
*A, manubrium; B, xyphoid, C; skin incision*

After subcutaneous and muscular preparation, the fourth or fifth intercostal space is chosen to open the parietal pleura with an incision that should exceed the length of the skin incision, particularly towards the back, to reduce the risk of costal fractures. For LITA harvesting, a retractor lifting the cranial rib should be used to improve LITA exposure.

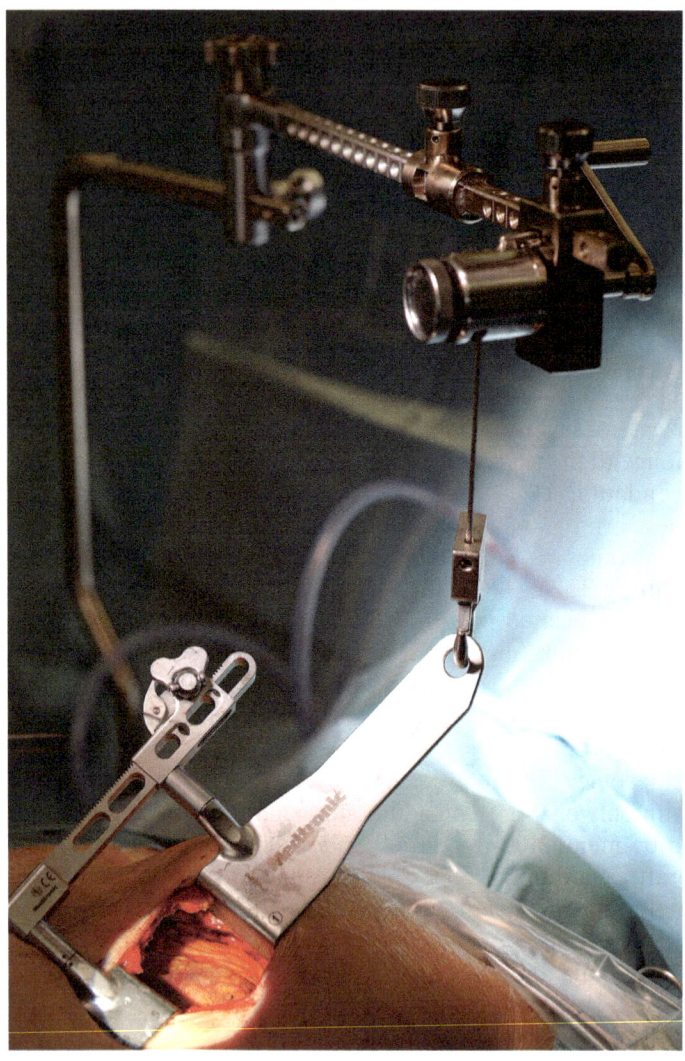

Photo 3.27: Lifting retractor for LITA harvesting (Thoratrak, Medtronic, Dublin, Ireland; Skyhook, Rultract Inc., Cleveland, OH, USA)

In order to allow for double lung ventilation during the operation, which is particularly important in patients with poor pulmonary function or in long-lasting multivessel operations, the pulmonary-fan technique can be applied: Cutting through the mediastinal pleura, the pericardium is incised 1–2 cm anterior of the phrenic nerve, and 8–12 sutures are stitched along the pericardio-pleural margin, carefully avoiding damage to the phrenic nerve. All suture ends are collected and pulled through the third or fourth intercostal space close to the midaxillary line, creating a fan that partially retracts the left lung and thus allows for double lung ventilation without impairment of LITA harvesting or anastomoses generation.

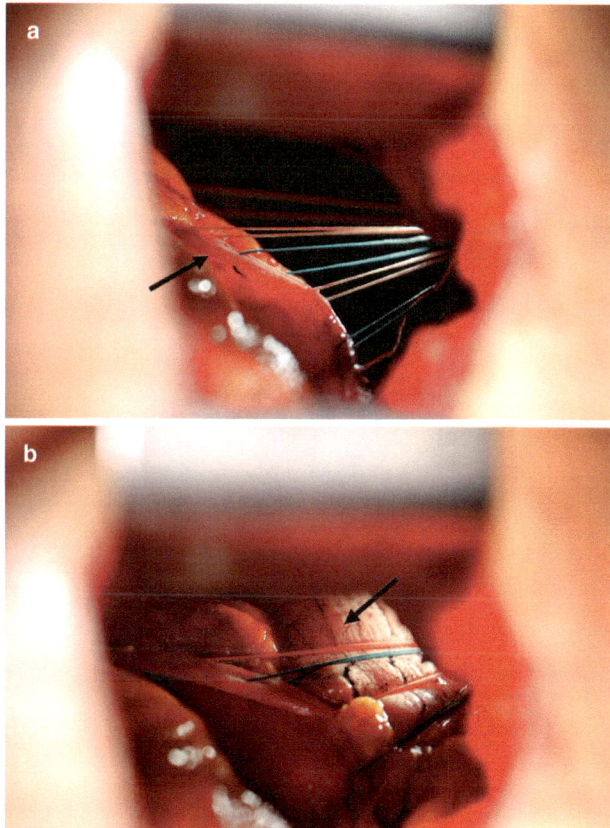

PHOTO 3.28A+B: Pulmonary-fan technique for double lung ventilation
*a: →, pericardio-pleural margin*
*b: →, ventilated lung*

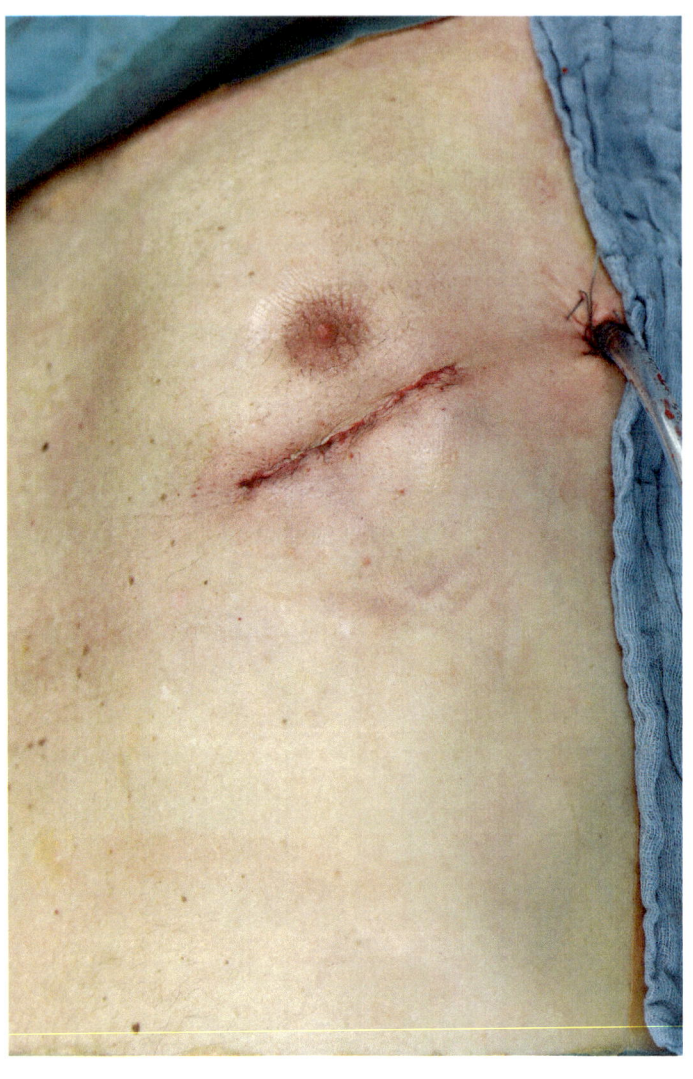

PHOTO 3.29: Cosmetic result after MIDCAB

## 3.3   Epiaortic Ultrasound

After sternotomy or left anterolateral thoracotomy, epiaortic ultrasound imaging is strongly recommended to assess the amount of atherosclerotic burden of the ascending aorta. This easy-to-use technique provides crucial information particularly with regard to central aortic anastomoses or aortic cannulation and clamping for CPB operations. Performing epiaortic ultrasound imaging at the beginning of the operation enables early and safe planning of the primary surgical technique as well as potential fallback options.

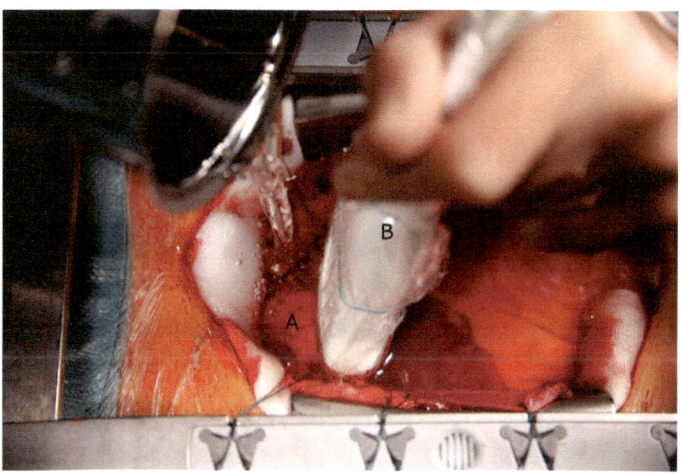

Photo 3.30: Epiaortic ultrasound imaging
A, ascending aorta; B, linear ultrasound probe

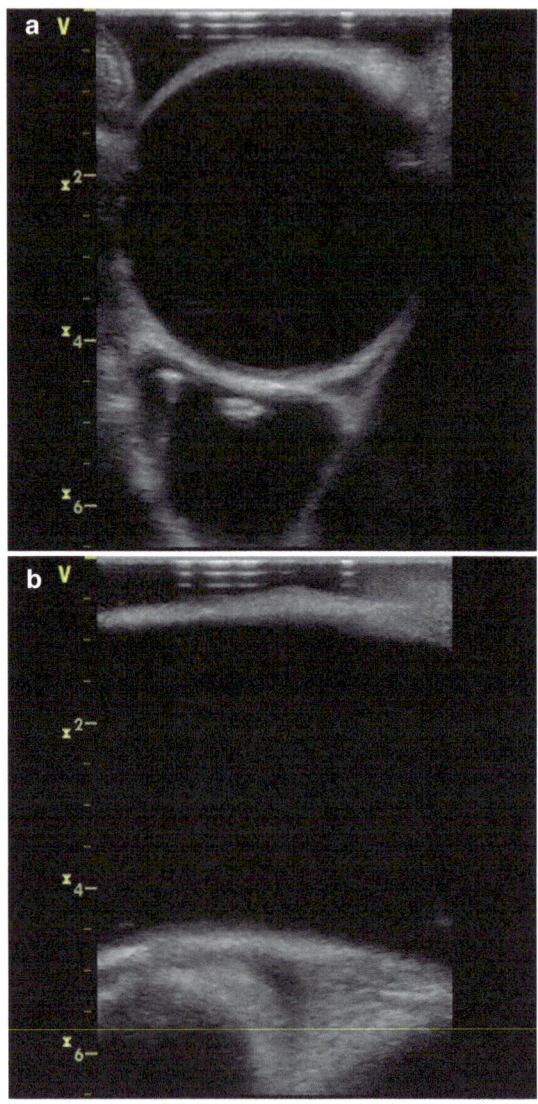

Photo 3.31a+b: Epiaortic ultrasound images of a non-atheromatous aorta
*a: Cross section*
*b: Longitudinal section*

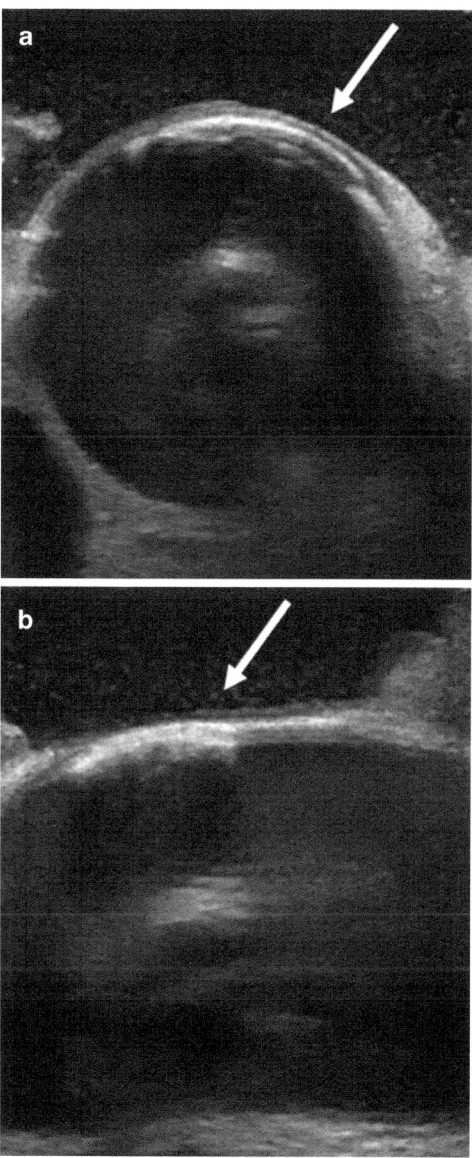

PHOTO 3.32A+B:  Epiaortic ultrasound images of a calcified aorta
*a: Cross section; →, plaque*
*b: Longitudinal section; →, plaque*

# 3.4    Intrathoracic Preparation

## 3.4.1    Off-Pump Preparation

For off-pump procedures, we recommend anticoagulation with initially 200 IU/kg intravenous heparin (target activated clotting time >300 s) after graft harvesting. Since the therapeutic effect of heparin decreases rapidly, frequent monitoring of the activated clotting time is necessary. For safety reasons, notable authorities in OPCAB surgery recommend target values >400 s.

The techniques for exposure of the cardiac wall areas to be revascularized depend on the type of thoracic access (OPCAB via sternotomy versus MIDCAB or MV-MICS via left anterolateral mini-thoracotomy), and therefore, are described in the following sub-chapters.

For cardiac displacement, positioning and target vessel exposure, apically suctioning positioner devices and suction stabilizers should be used, and are also available as MICS versions which we recommend particularly in cases of complex exposure. Additionally, we recommend pericardial traction sutures and a deep pericardial sling. In order to cope with bleeding from the target vessel during stitching, a carbon dioxide blower is recommended, whereas it should be used restrictively to avoid potential air embolism or damage to the vessel walls.

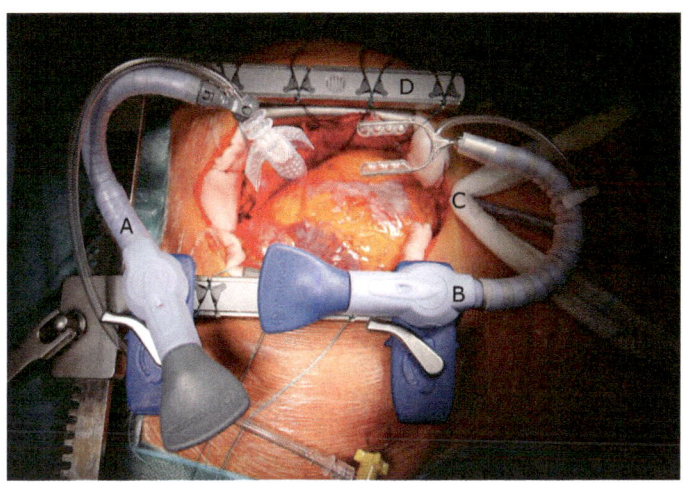

PHOTO 3.33:  Prepared off-pump setting after sternotomy
*A, apically suctioning positioner device (Starfish, Medtronic, Dublin, Ireland); B, suction stabilizer (Octopus, Medtronic, Dublin, Ireland); C, deep pericardial sling; D, sternal retractor (OctoBase, Medtronic, Dublin, Ireland) with pericardial traction sutures*

### 3.4.1.1   Cardiac Positioning After Sternotomy

After median sternotomy, we recommend insertion of a sternal retractor rotated by 180° to facilitate access particularly to the lateral and posterior target vessels.

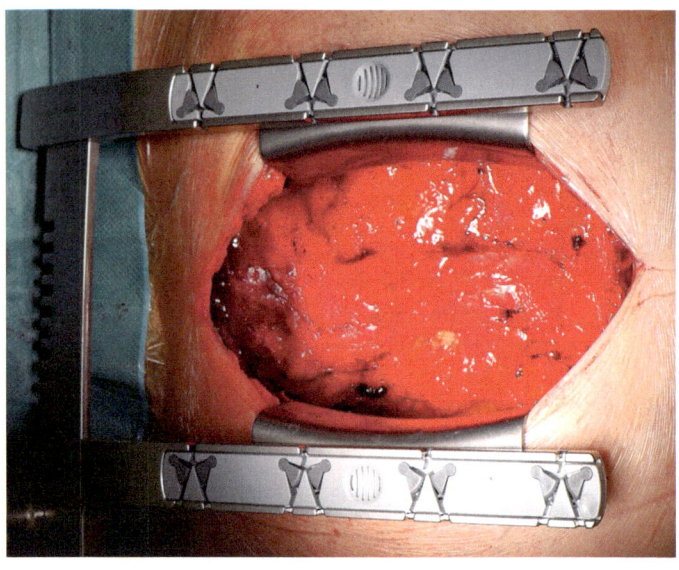

Photo 3.34: Sternal retractor rotated by 180°
*(OctoBase, Medtronic, Dublin, Ireland)*

Median pericardiotomy originates from the distal ascending aorta towards the diaphragm, and is rectangularly extended to the left towards the cardiac apex.

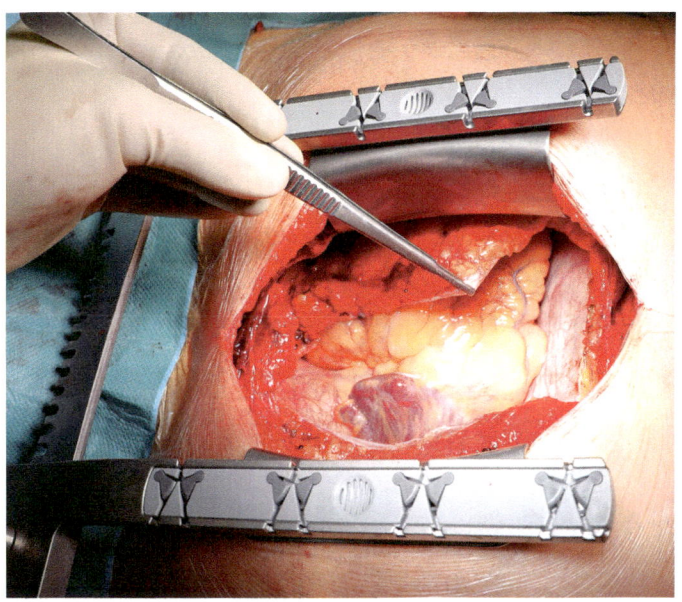

Photo 3.35: Rectangular pericardiotomy towards the cardiac apex

Lateral pericardial sutures are placed at both pericardiotomy margins, whereas the right-sided sutures should not pulled in order to allow the heart to move towards the right side during later enucleation. Additional deep lateral pericardial sutures on the left side support exposure of the anterior wall. These sutures should be stitched in a distance of at least 1 cm from the phrenic nerve.

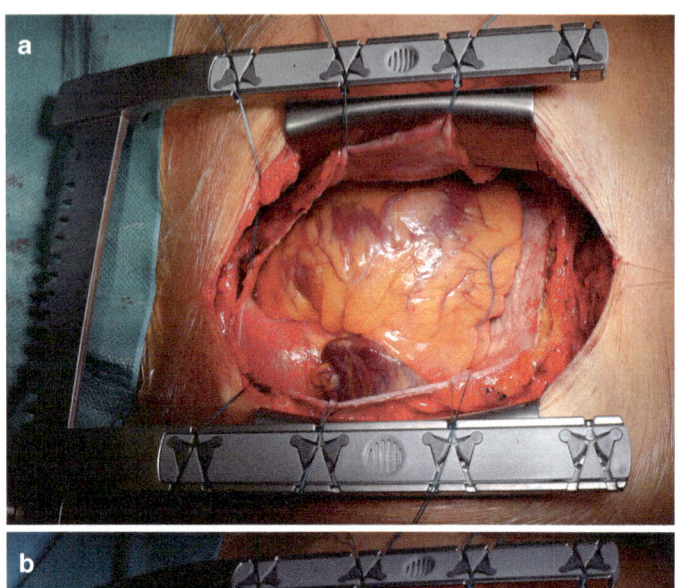

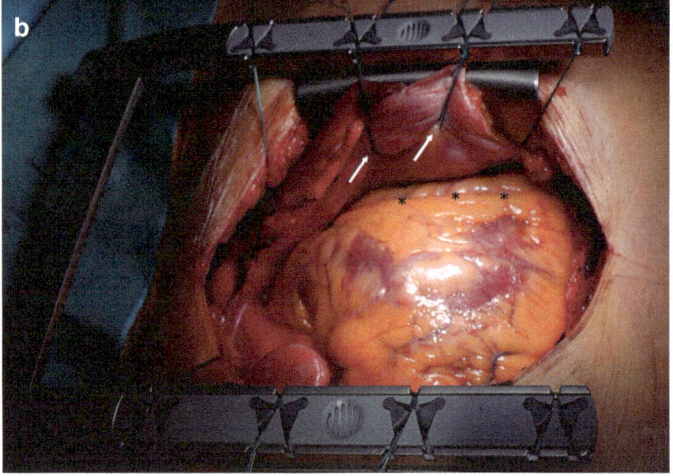

PHOTO 3.36A+B:  Lateral pericardial sutures
*Pericardial traction sutures at the pericardial margins.*
*Pericardial traction sutures at the pericardial margins, and addition-
ally deep on the left side. *, LAD; →, deep pericardial traction sutures.*

A technique very supportive in terms of cardiac enucle-ation is the positioning of a deep pericardial sling, consisting of a strong monofilament suture (such as 2-0) with down-snared moistened gauze placed as deep as possible in the oblique sinus close to the right lower pulmonary vein. Optimized positioning of this so-called "deep stitch" is an important prerequisite for successful enucleation of the heart. Anchoring the gauze sling too far on the left side, is a frequent mistake that can cause haemodynamic instability, and therefore enhances the risk of conversion to CPB.

In most cases, we recommend to conduct this so-called "deep stitch" not before completion of the revascularization on the anterior wall to achieve improved haemodynamic sta-bilization before this procedure. Optimized cardiac preload, supported by an operation table position with leg raise (ensure that soft pillars are laterally mounted to the opera-tion table preventing the legs from falling down), is essential before enucleation. This is one of the multiple moments dur-ing off-pump surgery that requires close communication between the surgeon and the anaesthesiologist. In order to keep the moment of cardiac manipulation as short and hae-modynamically negligible as possible, all required materials should be thoroughly prepared including a sucker in the hands of the attentive assistant.

At first, the heart is manually enucleated in a gentle man-ner exposing the oblique sinus. The sucker is used to exert tension on the dorsal pericardium close to the right lower pulmonary vein in order to allow for rapid stitching of the pericardium with the monofilament suture.

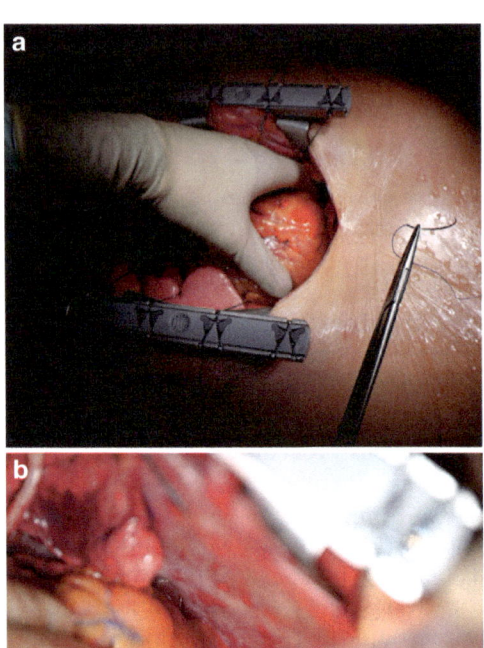

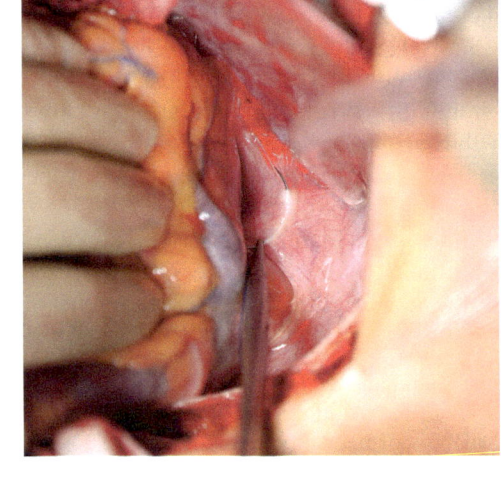

Photo 3.37a+b: Deep stitch
*The heart is manually enucleated (a), the sucker is used to exert tension on the dorsal pericardium (b), and the monofilament suture is stitched (b).*

The pericardially fixed sling suture is used to create a tourniquet for a longitudinally unfolded moistened gauze that is guided through the sling suture. The moistened gauze is positioned at the dorsal pericardium, and the tourniquet is tightened fixing the gauze to the pericardium.

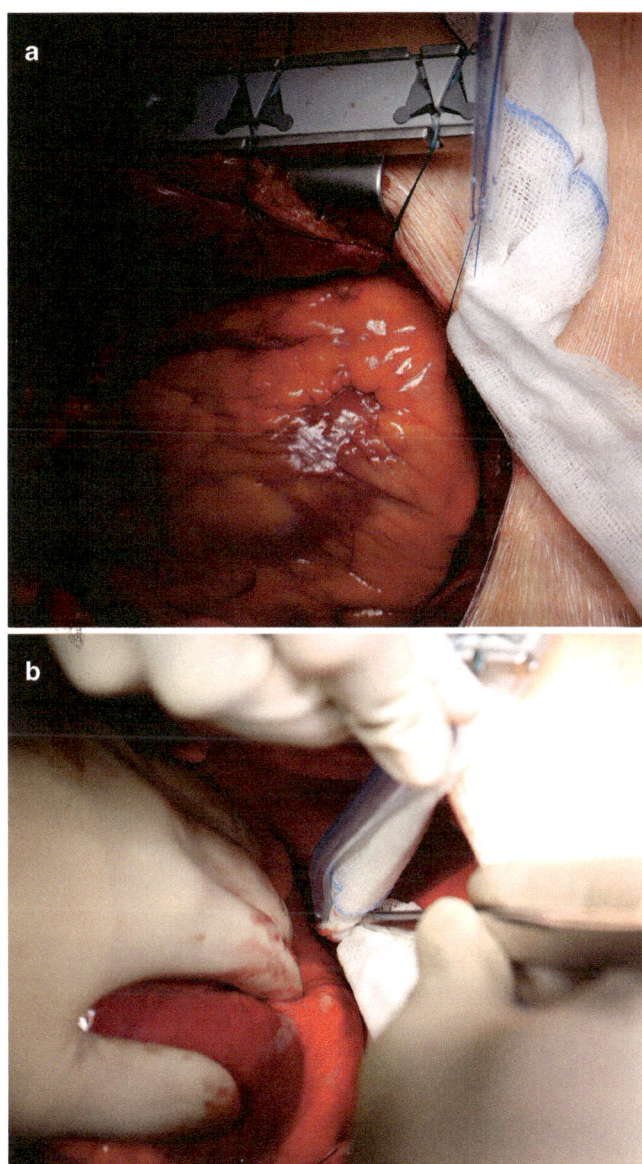

PHOTO 3.38A+B: Pericardial sling installation
*A moistened gauze is fixed to the dorsal pericardium applying the "deep stitch" sling suture.*

By pulling the lateral pericardial traction sutures and the two ends of the deep sling gauze, the heart is slowly enucleated to expose the lateral or the posterior wall. Again, the haemodynamics have to be carefully monitored and optimized.

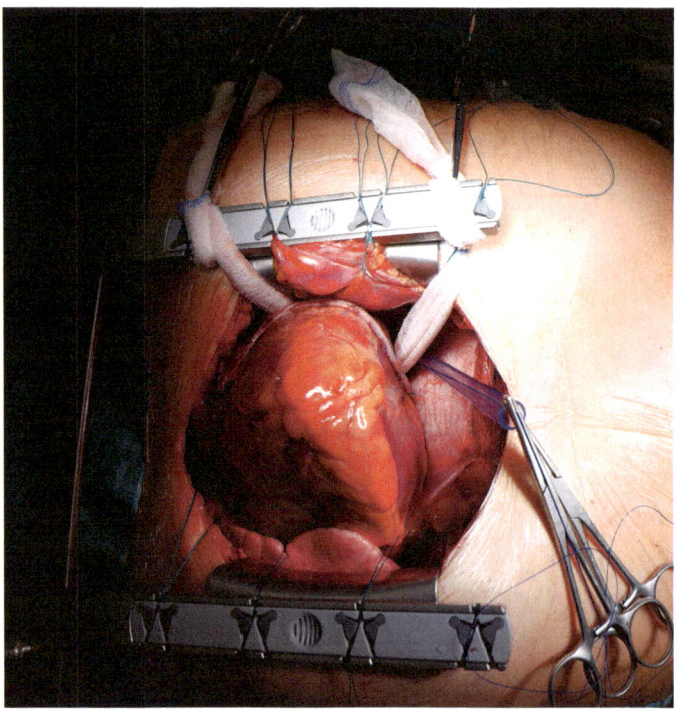

Photo 3.39: Cardiac enucleation by pericardial sutures and the deep sling

Additionally, an apically suctioning positioner device can be used to displace the heart as necessary while stabilizing the cardiac geometry (avoiding longitudinal "slumping down" of the heart) during enucleation, and to improve the target vessel access.

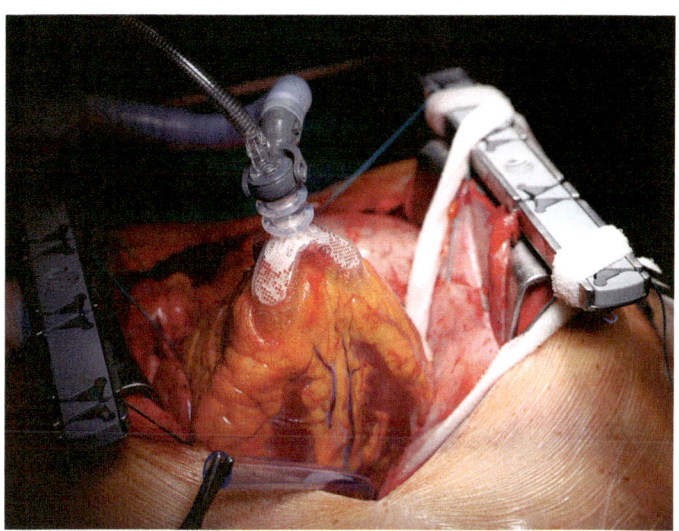

Photo 3.40: Cardiac enucleation supported by an apically suctioning positioner device
*(Starfish, Medtronic, Dublin, Ireland)*

For target vessel exposure, a suction stabilizer device is applied, whereby the stabilizer arms should be thoroughly shaped according to the geometry of the cardiac surface, and holes may be occluded by bone wax to prevent coronary side branches from suctioning.

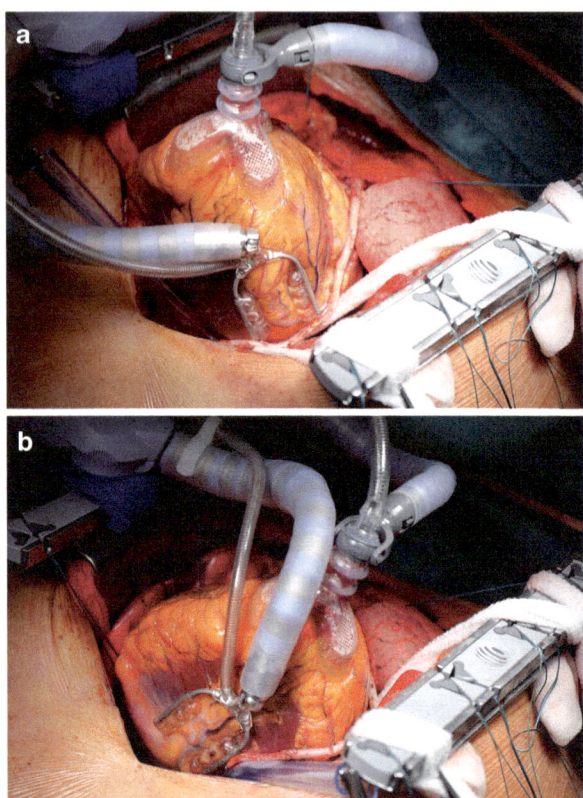

PHOTO 3.41A+B: Target vessel exposure by a suction stabilizer device Coronary artery exposure on the lateral (a) and posterior (b) wall. *(Octopus, Medtronic, Dublin, Ireland)*

### 3.4.1.2    Cardiac Positioning After Left Anterolateral Mini-Thoracotomy

*Positioning for Central Anastomoses to the Aorta*

For aortic anastomoses, the pericardial incision is caudally extended to the right, and the operation table is rotated to the same side.

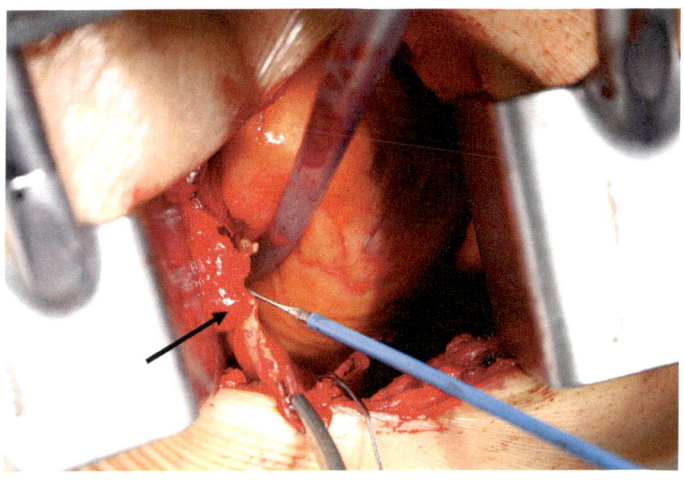

PHOTO 3.42: Pericardial incision to the right
→, *caudal incision of the pericardium*

Serial lateral pericardial sutures are placed on the right side and pulled to lift the aorta and move it towards left.

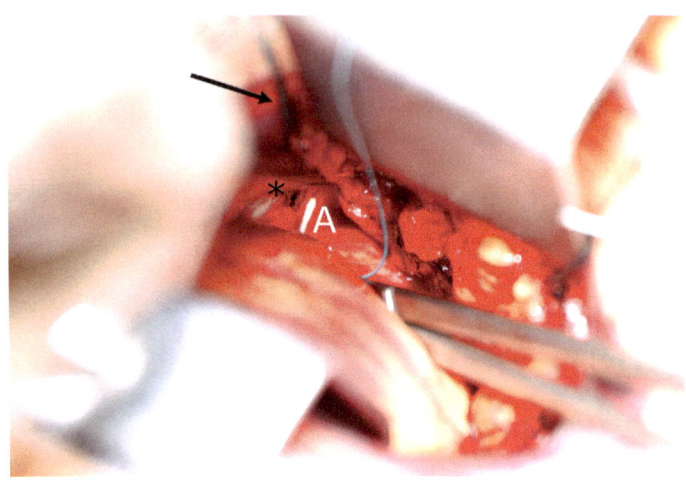

PHOTO 3.43:  Pericardial sutures
→, *pulled lateral pericardial suture; *, left pericardial margin; A, needle of the next lateral pericardial suture*

In order to further improve this motion, a moistened gauze can be placed between the aorta and the right pericardium, which additionally can be used to avoid a prolapse of the right atrial appendix.

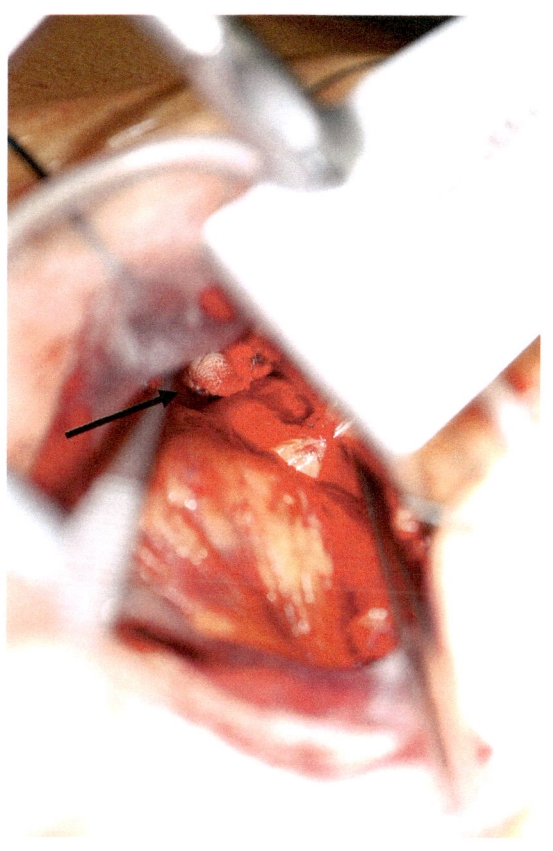

PHOTO 3.44: Gauze placed between aorta and right pericardium
→, *gauze;* *, *aorta*

Furthermore, the pulmonary end-expiratory pressure can be enhanced to move the aorta towards the thoracotomy. The suction stabilizer is used to gently press down the pulmonary artery.

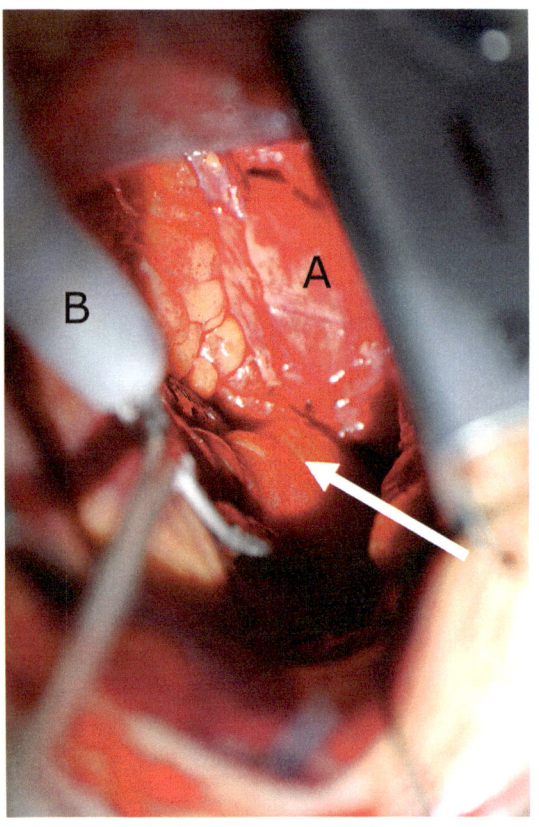

PHOTO 3.45: Installation of the suction stabilizer
→, *pulmonary artery; A, aorta; B, suction stabilizer*

Afterwards, a central anastomotic device can be inserted into the aorta. Alternatively, the aorta may be clamped tangentially. Both techniques should be used only after exclusion of local atherosclerosis. Therefore, we perform preoperative computed tomography scanning and intraoperative epiaortic ultrasound imaging in all patients who undergo MV-MICS.

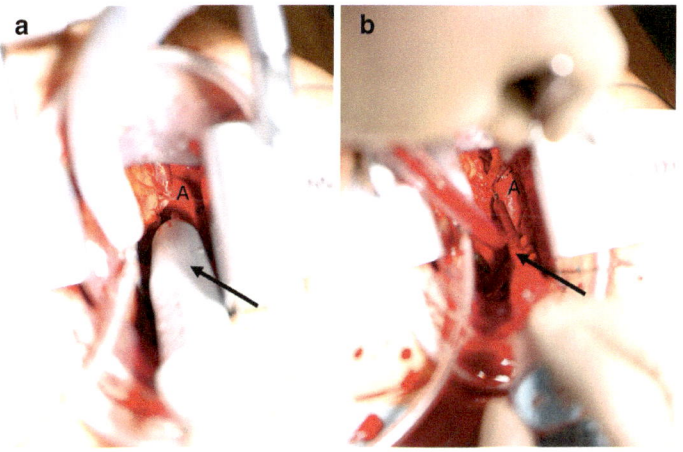

PHOTO 3.46A+B:   Insertion of the central anastomotic device (Heart String, Getinge, Gothenburg, Sweden)
→, *central anastomotic device; A, aorta*

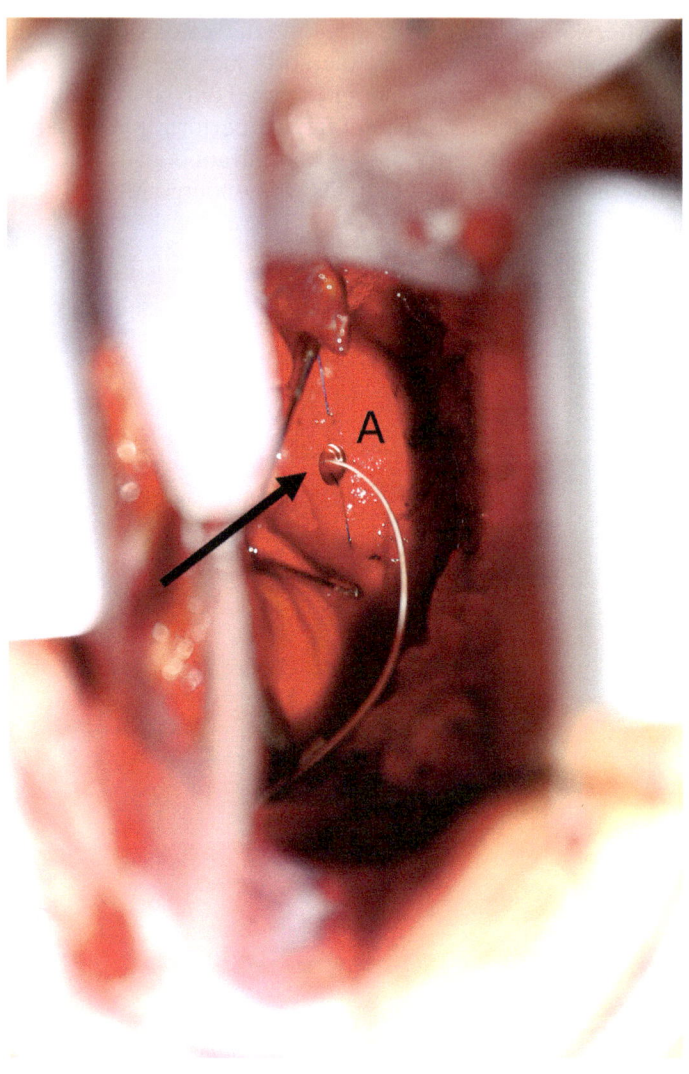

PHOTO 3.47: Inserted anastomotic device
→, *inserted anastomotic device; A, aorta*

The pulmonary-fan technique described above can be applied to allow double-lung ventilation also during generation of an aortic anastomosis.

*Positioning for Central Anastomoses of Composite Grafts*

For composite T- and Y-graft anastomoses, the LITA is exposed by usage of a suction stabilizer (without activated suction), optionally equipped with a soft and wet cover, such as a moistened gauze. The stabilizer is positioned in low distance to the cardiac surface, and the LITA is orthogonally loaded onto the stabilizer, and optionally fixed with a suture.

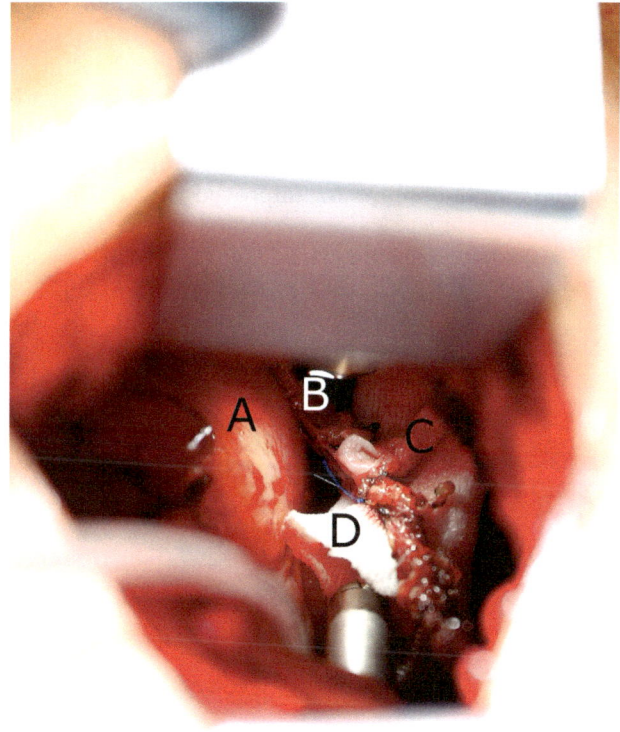

Photo 3.48: Usage of suction stabilizer for composite T- or Y-graft anastomoses
*A, aorta; B, LITA; C, SVG; D, suction stabilizer*

*Positioning for Peripheral Anastomoses*

In order to expose proximal segments of an OM, the heart is gently rotated in a counter-clockwise manner, and a suction stabilizer is applied to fix the position. Optionally, a suctioning positioner device can be used to displace and stabilize the luxated heart.

For exposure of the lateral and posterolateral wall, cardiac enucleation is conducted similarly to traditional OPCAB techniques: The pericardial incision is caudally extended to the right, and the operation table is rotated to the same side. The left pericardium is deeply incised in the area around the apex as well as next to the pulmonary artery, paying attention to the course of the phrenic nerve, to generate a semi-mobile pericardial flap that allows for improved view on the lateral wall.

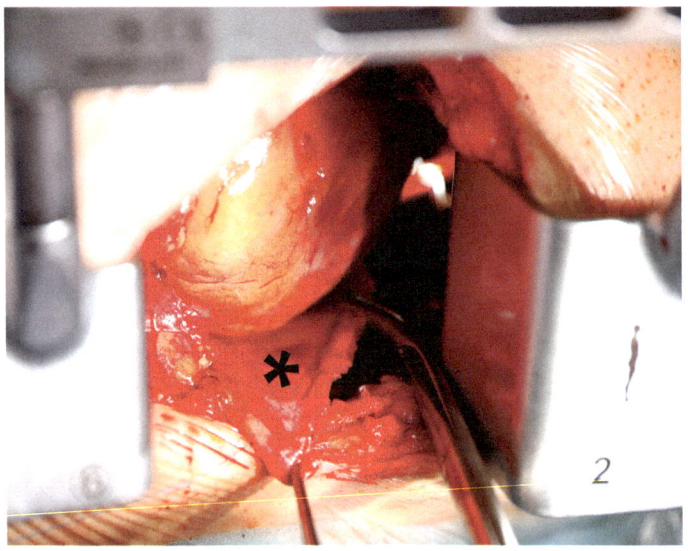

PHOTO 3.49: Left pericardial flap preparation
*, *prepared pericardial flap*

During short deflation of the lung, an armless suctioning positioner device, equipped with a traction suture, is used to modify the cardiac axis to expose the target coronary arteries. Afterwards, a suction stabilizer is utilized to fix the desired wall segment.

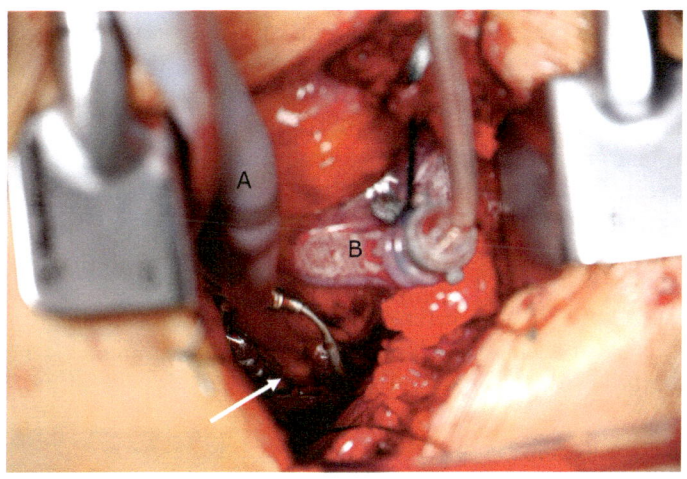

PHOTO 3.50: Exposure of the lateral wall
→, *exposure of OM; A, suction stabilizer; B, armless suctioning positioner device*

Aiming at PDA exposure, the heart is gently rotated in a clockwise manner, and a suction stabilizer is applied to fix the position without usage of a suctioning positioner device.

## 3.4.2   On-Pump Preparation

For on-pump procedures, we recommend anticoagulation with initially 300 IU/kg intravenous heparin (target activated clotting time >400 s) after graft harvesting. Median pericardiotomy from the distal ascending aorta to the cardiac apex is followed by lateral pericardial sutures. Arterial and venous cannulas are inserted into the distal ascending aorta and the right atrium or the venae cavae, respectively. Insertion position, angle and depth of the arterial cannula should be adapted according to the aortic geometry and the pattern of atherosclerotic plaques. In order to minimize haemodilution by CPB, antegrade or retrograde priming with autologous blood can be conducted. For cardioplegia delivery, antegrade administration via the ascending aorta and retrograde administration via the venous coronary sinus should be considered as well as additional administration via peripherally anastomosed bypasses during the course of the operation. Particularly in case of occluded or subtotally occluded coronary arteries, antegrade administration only may not suffice to guarantee complete myocardial protection during cardiac arrest. Left ventricular unloading by left atrial or left ventricular vent catheters should be considered especially in case of aortic valve regurgitation. For exposure of the lateral and inferior wall, a deep pericardial sling, such as for the off-pump procedures, or a moistened gauze surrounding the inferior vena cava can be positioned. Then, cross-clamping of the ascending aorta is followed by cardioplegia administration.

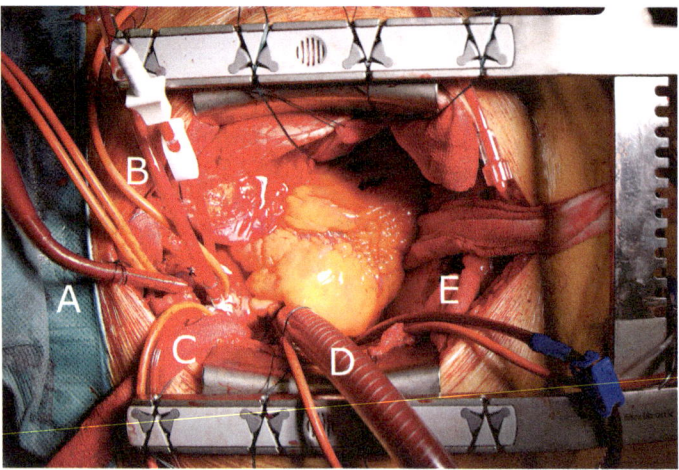

PHOTO 3.51: Prepared On-Pump Setting
*A, arterial cannula; B, antegrade cardioplegia catheter; C, left ventricular vent catheter; D, venous cannula; E, retrograde cardioplegia catheter*

# 3.5   Anastomoses

## 3.5.1   General Considerations

### 3.5.1.1   Equipment

For smooth and controlled stitching, a round handle micro-surgical needle holder is required. As anastomotic sutures, double needle polypropylene 7-0 or 8-0, in case of sclerotic vessel walls equipped with needles featuring increased strength and bend resistance, should be chosen.

In order to preserve the blood flow through the coronary vessel during off-pump procedures, and to facilitate safe and controlled stitching in off-pump as well as on-pump operations, coronary shunts should be inserted into all target vessels. Furthermore, additional shunt insertion into the bypass graft supports adequate stitching particularly around the heel of an end-to-side anastomosis and around the edges of a side-to-side anastomosis. The shunt size should be chosen large enough to avoid relevant bleeding, yet small enough not to damage a degenerated coronary vessel or impede adequate stitching if the shunt fits too tight.

### 3.5.1.2   Graft and Target Vessel Geometry

After pericardiotomy, the complete bypass graft architecture should be planned thoroughly. Besides appropriate length of each graft, positioning of the anastomoses is crucial. Branched, calcified or small-calibre (<1 mm) parts of the coronary arteries, or short plaque-free parts with relevant distal stenoses are no good candidates for anastomoses. Furthermore, competitive flow via not severely stenosed coronary arteries has to be considered, whereas in doubt, a properly sutured anastomosis should not compromise native coronary flow even in case of bypass occlusion, while the absence of a bypass may result in incomplete revascularization, particularly in case of future development or progress of stenoses.

When planning the anastomotic geometry, the target vessel side-incision size, the bypass end shape or side-incision size, the angle between graft and target vessel, and the surrounding epicardial tissue structure have to synergistically support the generation of a perfect anastomosis.

In case of orthogonal anastomoses (end-to-side or "diamond" shape side-to-side peripheral anastomoses, or T-shape central anastomoses), the length of a target vessel or bypass side incision should not exceed the diameter of the smaller vessel. Otherwise, if the incisions are chosen too long, the lumen of the smaller vessel will be flattened by lateral tension to the vascular walls, resulting in the "seagull" phenomenon for thin bypasses to thicker coronary arteries [1], or in the "inverted seagull" phenomenon for thick bypasses to thinner target vessels. While the first phenomenon becomes obvious at the latest at the end of the anastomosis, the "inverted seagull" issue may be masked under the thick bypass vessel, and thereby overlooked. As an alternative to short incisions, a long parallel incision into the thinner vessel can be generated if the other vessel is thick enough to allow for an oblique or even orthogonal incision, and in case of the oblique incision, the whole bypass geometry also allows for an oblique anastomosis Fig. 3.1.

If neither short incisions nor the latter solution are eligible, side-to-side anastomoses should be avoided. In this scenario, conventional end-to-side bypasses or "mini-T-grafts" can be sutured. Mini-T-grafts are particularly used in case of multiple arterial grafting with sequentially anastomosed composite grafts exhibiting small diameters. In order to avoid side-to-side anastomoses, mini-T-grafts from the composite bypass artery can be anastomosed to the target vessels in a parallel end-to-side manner.

In case of parallel anastomoses (end- or side-to-side peripheral anastomoses or Y-shape central anastomoses), longer incisions are possible. Incisions should be initiated with a microsurgical knife and extended by round handle micro-scissors. The end of a graft should be prepared by a curved cut that is extended at the heel. The distance between heel and toe should exceed the incision length of the other vessel, so that the graft does not present a flat profile in the anastomosis, but a "cobra head" shape.

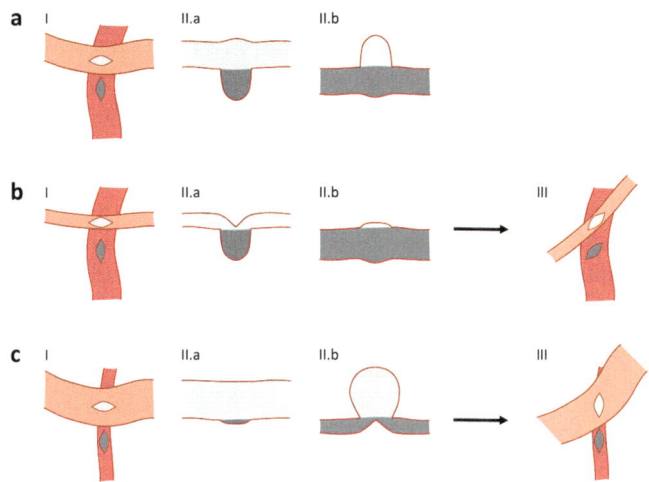

FIGURE 3.1 Side-to-side anastomoses in case of relevant size-mismatch

Side-to-side anastomoses between (**a**) vessels of equal size, (**b**) small-diameter bypass and large-diameter target vessel (resulting in the "seagull" phenomenon), and (**c**) large-diameter bypass and small target vessel (resulting in the "inverted seagull" phenomenon)

Target vessel: Red wall and dark-grey lumen; Bypass vessel: Orange wall and light-grey lumen

**I**, size relation between bypass and target vessel; **II**, side views of the sutured anastomosis displaying the remaining lumina of both vessels from two viewing directions (**II.a** and **II.b**) showing each of the vessels from a parallel as well as an orthogonal point of view; **III**, solutions for longer incisions with oblique direction in the thicker vessels and additionally oblique geometry of the anastomosis

Regarding the anastomosis angle between target vessel and bypass, large angles between 45° and 90° should be avoided, since unfavourable flow dynamics and the risk of graft kinking may impede the bypass durability, particularly in case of orthogonal side-to-side anastomoses. In order to avoid graft kinking, the surrounding epicardial tissue has to be adequately prepared, especially if the target vessel has an intramural location or is enclosed by fat tissue.

In case of on-pump surgery, utmost care has to be taken of the appropriate lengths and geometry of the bypasses, since the anastomoses are generated on a collapsed heart. In this context, thorough measurements before cardiac unloading by the heart-lung machine are helpful.

The sequence of bypass grafting in off-pump procedures can support hemodynamic stabilization of the patient during the further course of the operation. In this context, primary revascularization on the anterior wall before enucleation of the heart and early revascularization of critically stenosed coronary arteries may be even mandatory to allow for hemodynamic stability during further parts of the operation.

### 3.5.1.3   Stitching

Precise stitching begins with correct positioning of the needle in the needle holder. Ideally, the surgeon's hands stay in the same relaxed position, stabilized at the margins of the thoracic retractor, for all stitches. In the chapter "needle holder management", correct positioning of the needle in the needle holder is depicted for anastomoses on the anterior wall as well as on the posterior and lateral walls. The needle position has to allow for radial stitching so that the vessel walls are always passed through in a 90° angle, stitching at first through the intima of the target vessels, which avoids intima or media delamination in diseased coronary arteries. The distance between stitch hole and margin of the vessel incision or graft end has to be equal for all stitches. The distance between two stitches should be constant for both vessels, except for end-to-side anastomoses, in which the distances at the toe of the graft should exceed the corresponding distances at the target vessel to generate the "cobra head" shape. In any case, final de-airing should not be forgotten.

## 3.5.2   Central Bypass Anastomoses

Central bypass anastomoses can be sewn directly to the aorta, or to other bypasses resulting in composite grafts. For central anastomoses of composite grafts in off-pump procedures, stabilization tools facilitate precise and rapid stitching.

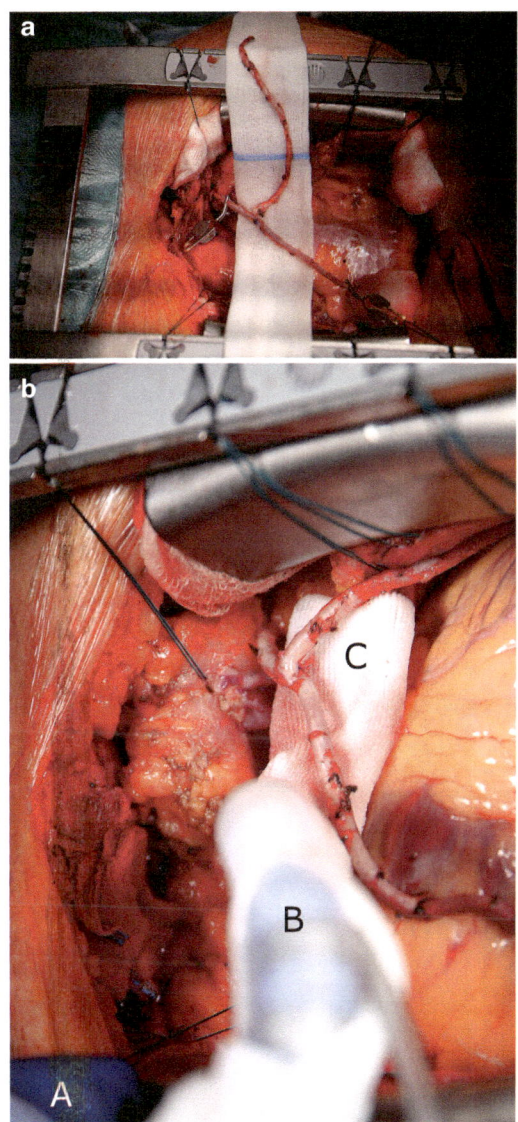

PHOTO 3.52A+B:  a: Vessel stabilization 1
*"Hammock" gauze sponge*
b: Vessel stabilization 2
*Off-pump tissue stabilizer platform. A, suction stabilizer; B, arm of*
*the suction stabilizer; C, T-graft anastomosis on stabilization platform*

### 3.5.2.1   Composite T- and Y-Grafts

After calculation of the bypass architecture, the central graft
is proximally clamped and longitudinally incised. Afterwards,
the central end of the peripheral graft is shaped. Optionally,
shunts can be inserted.

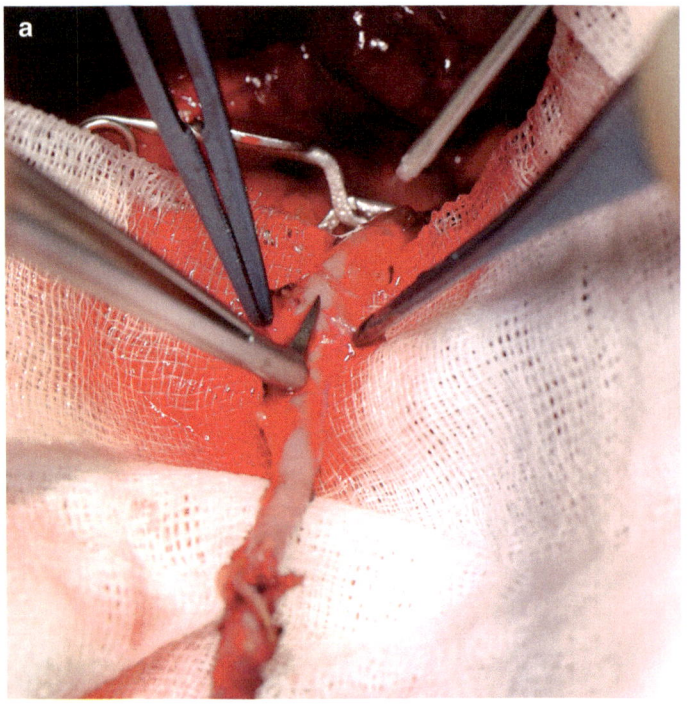

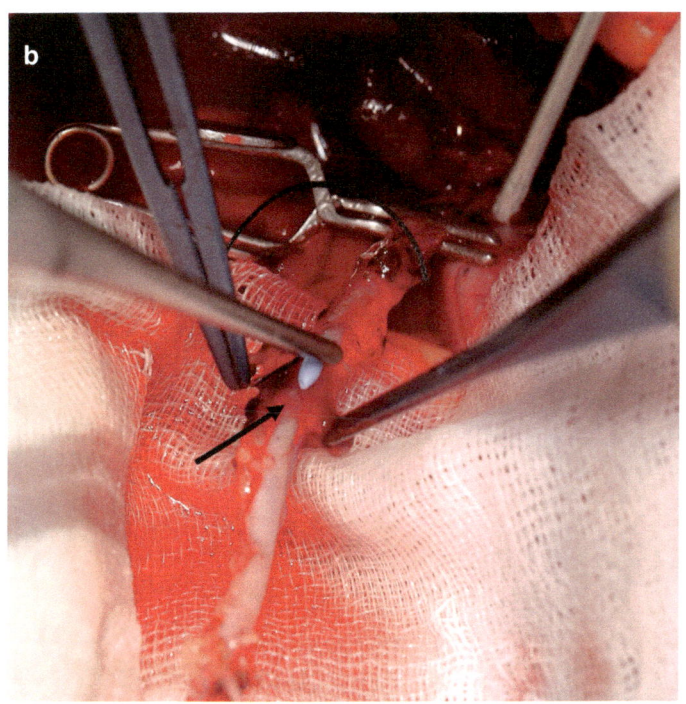

PHOTO 3.53A+B:  a: Graft preparation
*Graft preparation on a "Hammock" gauze sponge*
b: Shunt insertion
→, *unt*

The first stitches can be placed either at the heel of the peripheral graft or at the position directly in opposite to the surgeon. Starting from there, both needles are used to complete the anastomosis. Alternatively, only one needle can be used to generate the anastomosis, avoiding a change of the stitching direction of the running suture. Depending on the wall stability of both vessels, a few initial stitches may be considered to be performed in a "parachute" technique.

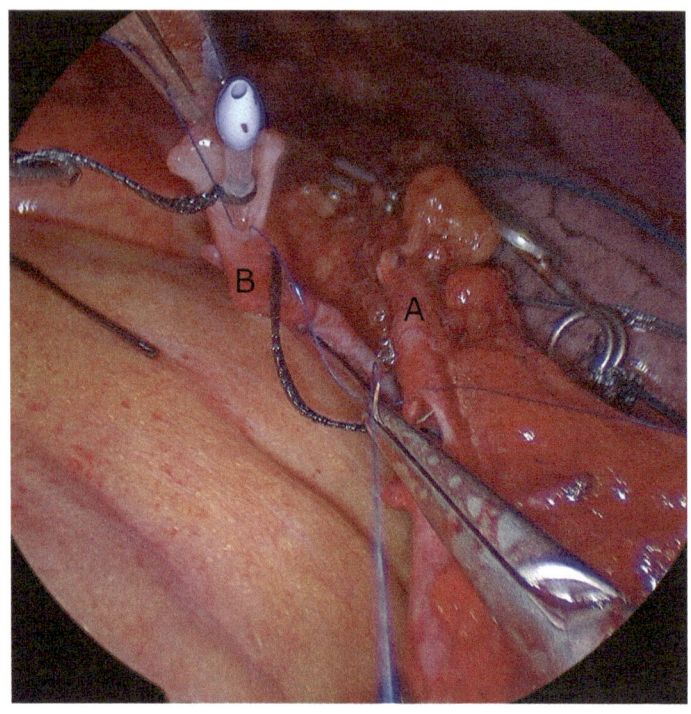

PHOTO 3.54:  Initial parachute stitches
*A, LITA; B, RITA*

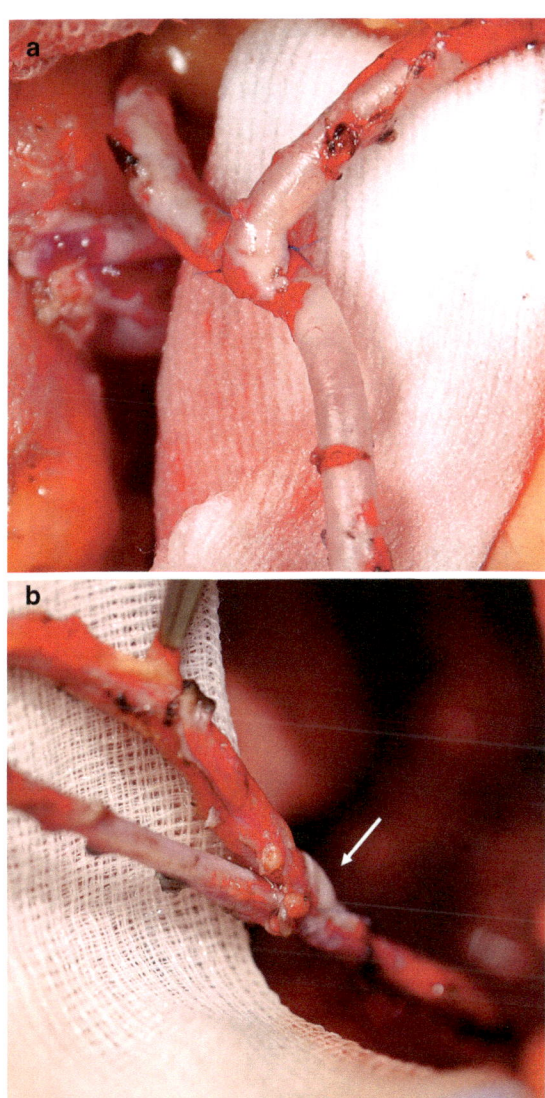

PHOTO 3.55A+B:  a: Completed anastomosis—T-graft
*Completed central T-shape anastomosis resembling a "cobra head"*
b: Completed anastomosis—Y-graft
→, *Y-shape anastomosis*

### 3.5.2.2   Aortic Anastomoses

In off-pump procedures, anastomotic devices should be used to avoid aortic clamping.

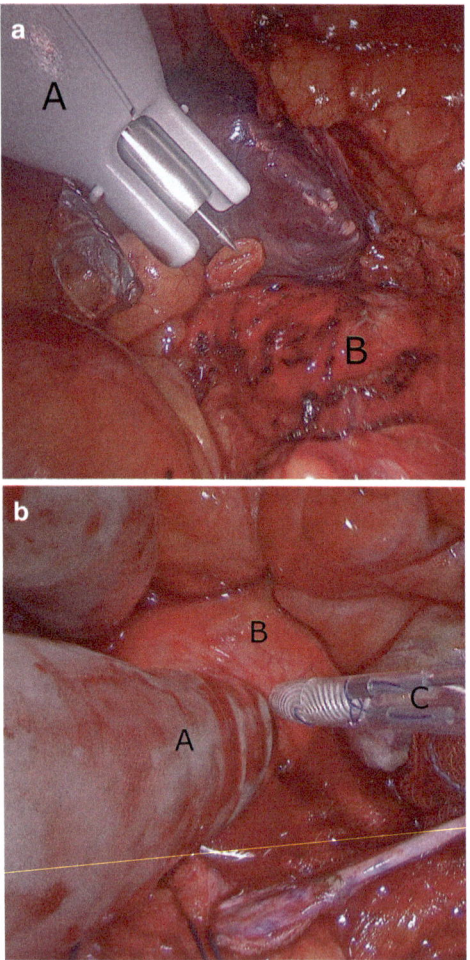

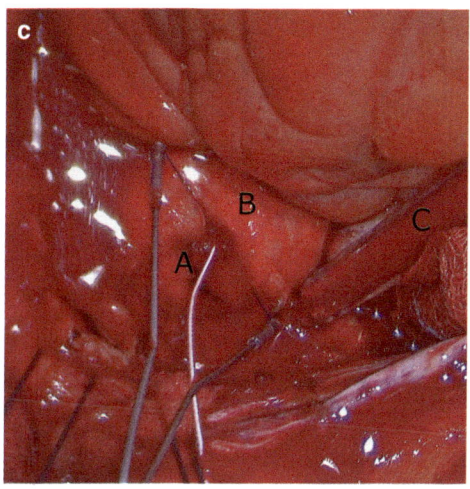

PHOTO 3.56A–C:  a: Clampless anastomotic device insertion 1
*A, puncture device; B, aorta*
b: Clampless anastomotic device insertion 2
*A, finger on top of the punched hole in the aorta; B, aorta; C, anasto-*
*motic device*
c: Installed clampless anastomotic device
*A, hole for the bypass anastomosis; B, aorta; C, cell saver sucker*

After calculation of the bypass length, the central end of the graft is shaped. Optionally, a shunt can be inserted.

The first stitches can be placed either at the heel of the graft or at the position directly in opposite to the surgeon. Starting from there, both needles are used to complete the anastomosis, whereat in most cases, the aortic wall should be stitched perforating the intima at first. Alternatively, only one needle can be used to generate the anastomosis, avoiding a change of the stitching direction of the running suture. Depending on the wall stability of both vessels, a few initial stitches may be considered to be performed in a "parachute" technique.

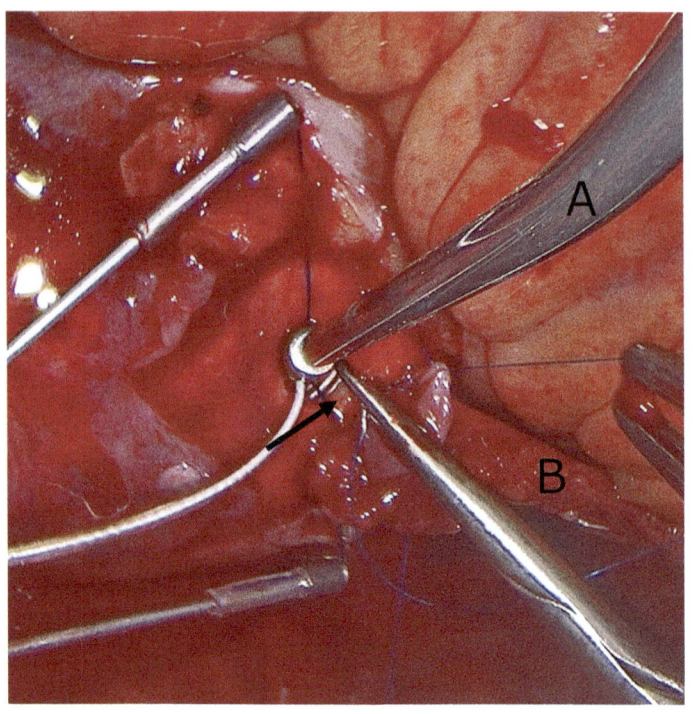

PHOTO 3.57: Parachute stitches
→, *parachute stitches; A, blood sucker; B, bypass graft*

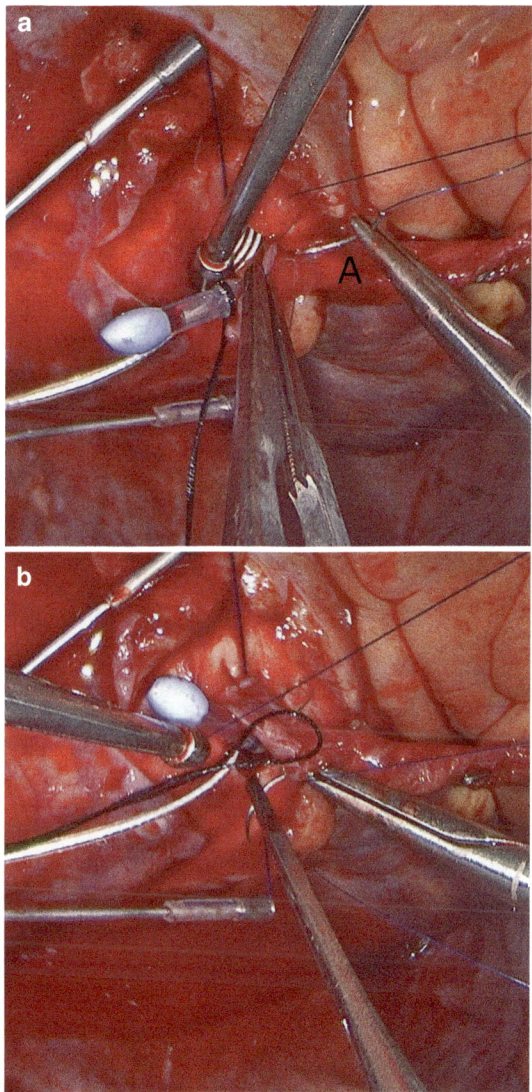

PHOTO 3.58A+B: a: Surrounding stitches 1
*Surrounding stitches with inserted shunt in the bypass graft (A)*
b: Surrounding stitches 2
*Surrounding stitches with inserted shunt in the bypass graft*

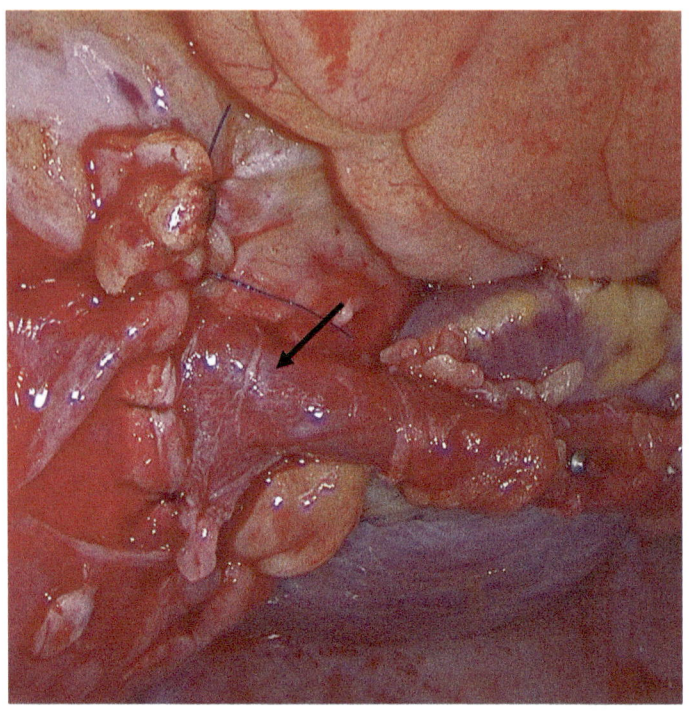

Photo 3.59: Completed anastomosis
→, *Completed central aortic anastomosis resembling a "cobra head"*

### 3.5.3 Peripheral Bypass Anastomoses

#### 3.5.3.1 Target Vessel Preparation

For exposure of the target coronary artery, all covering tissue layers have to be carefully dissected, which may include epicardium, epicardial fat tissue, and myocardium.

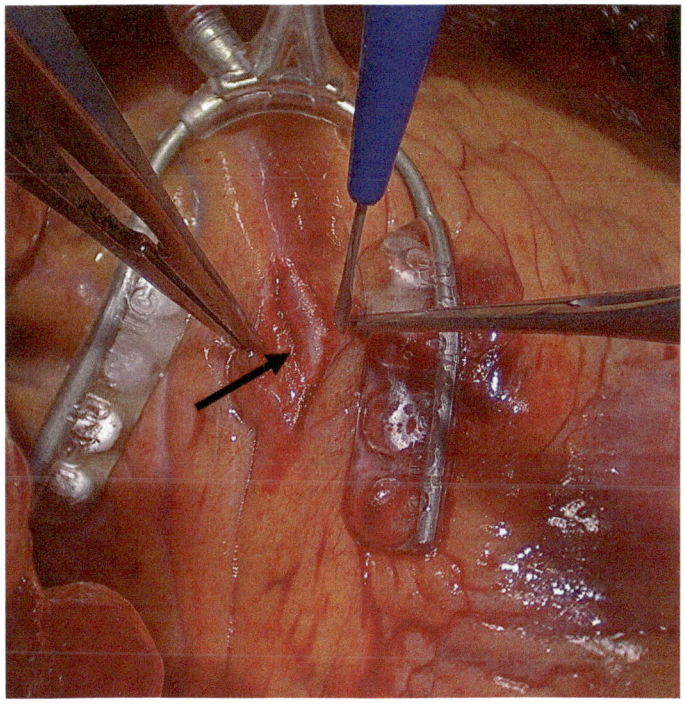

PHOTO 3.60: Tissue dissection
→, *target coronary artery (in this case: LAD)*

On both sides of the coronary artery, tissue-everting sutures (polypropylene 6–0) are stitched.

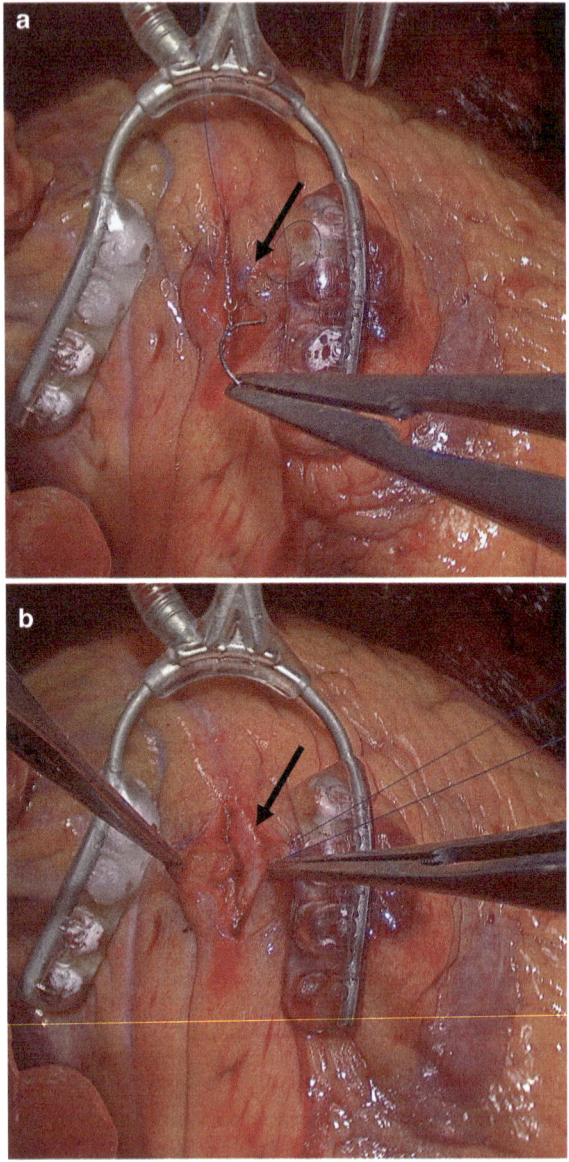

PHOTO 3.61A+B: Tissue-everting sutures
*a: →, tissue-everting suture*
*b: →, target coronary artery with one tissue-everting suture*

In order to stop bleeding after subsequent incision, a soft tourniquet-equipped suture (polypropylene 4–0) for vessel occlusion is placed around the coronary artery directly proximally (or distally—in case of proximally occluded while distally collateralized arteries) of the planned incision site.

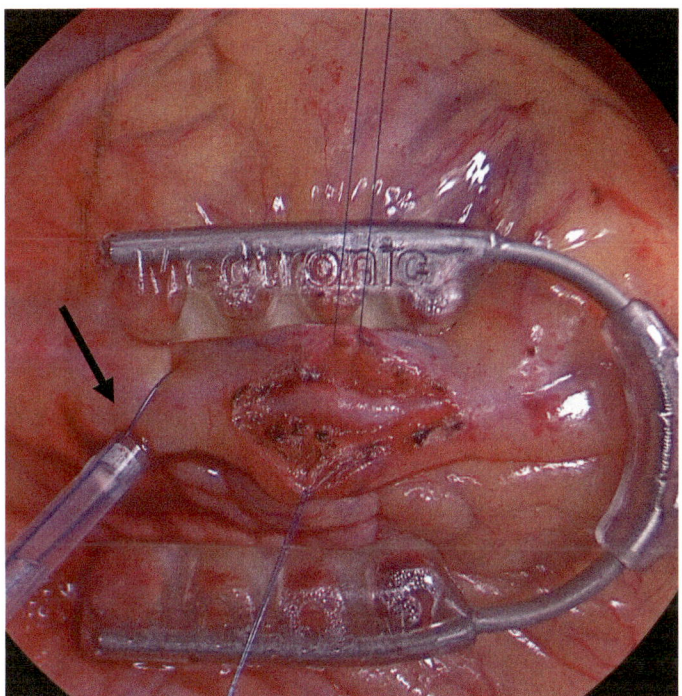

PHOTO 3.62: Proximal vessel occlusion
→, *proximal vessel occlusion*

The coronary artery is longitudinally incised, and the tourniquet suture is tightened immediately. Shortly loosening the tourniquet suture allows for estimation of the native blood flow through the coronary artery.

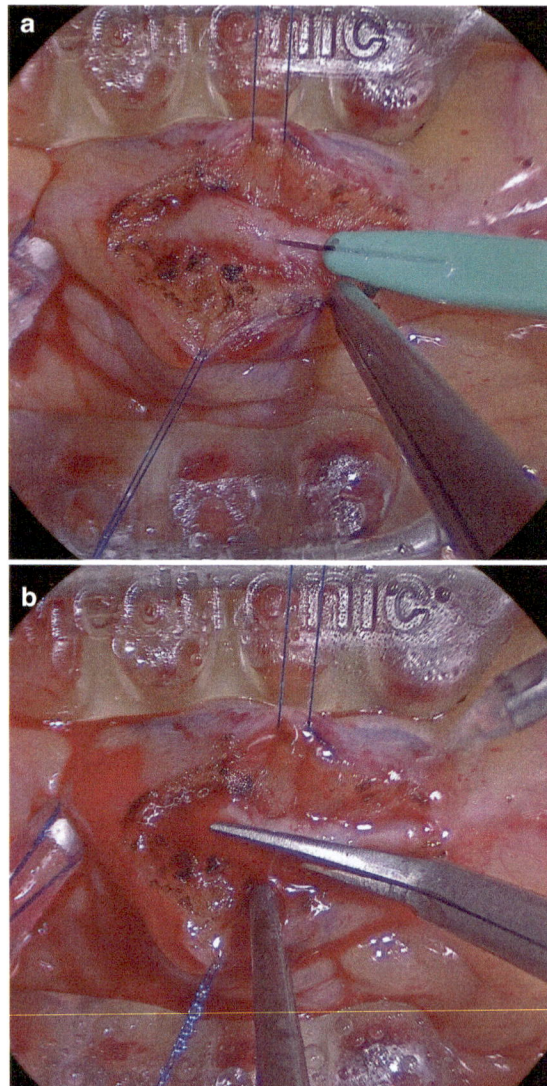

PHOTO 3.63A+B: Vessel incision
*a: Incision with a sharp scalpel*
*b: Longitudinal incision of the coronary artery*

A coronary shunt is inserted with its longer end towards the vessel inflow direction and its shorter end manipulated towards the outflow direction. Depending on the geometry of the vessel and particularly its side branches, the ideal shunt direction may vary. Afterwards, the tourniquet suture is loosened.

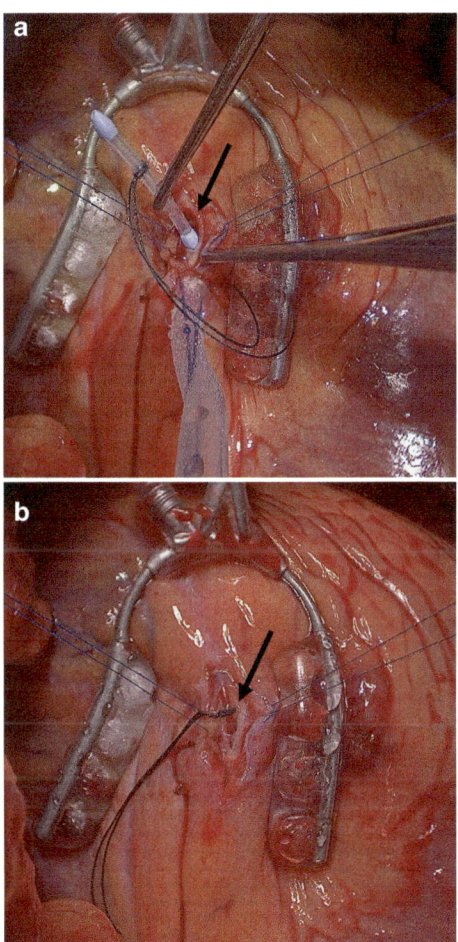

Photo 3.64a+b: Shunt insertion
*a: →, procedure of insertion*
*b: →, correctly placed coronary shunt*

### 3.5.3.2    Needle Holder Management

When stitching peripheral bypass anastomoses, adequate needle holder management facilitates the process. Optimal positioning of the needle improves ergonomics, accuracy and speed of the operation (Figs. 3.2 and 3.3).

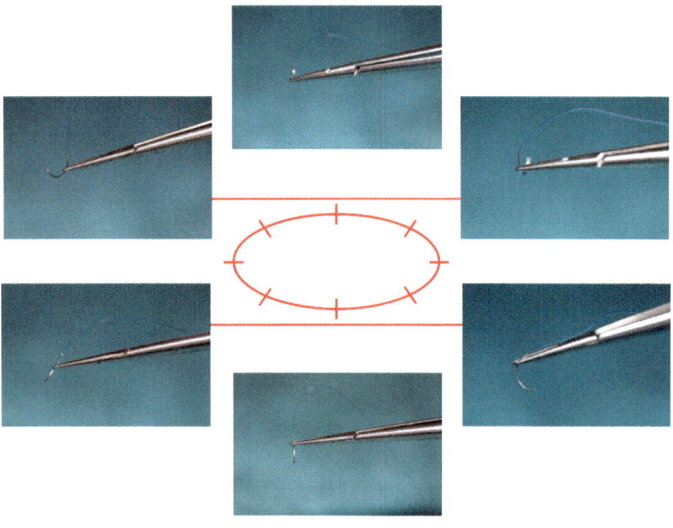

Figure 3.2: Needle holder management for anastomoses on the anterior wall

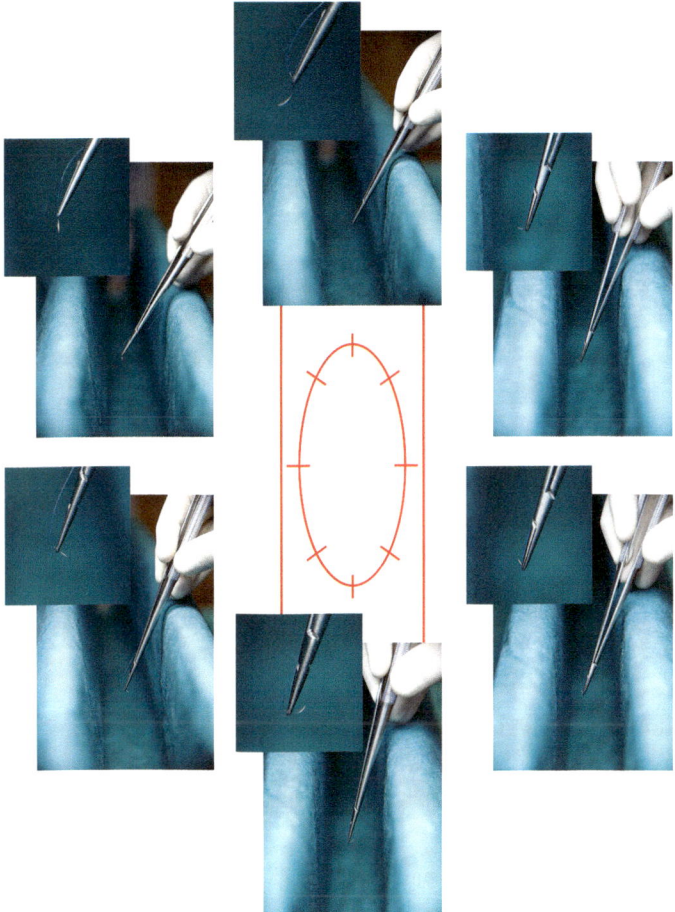

FIGURE 3.3: Needle holder management for anastomoses on the posterior and lateral walls

### 3.5.3.3 End-to-Side Anastomoses

End-to-side bypass anastomoses can be sutured in a parallel or an orthogonal fashion, depending on the planned bypass geometry. Common strategies for the start point of stitching include the heel of the bypass and the area most distant from the surgeon. Starting from there, both needles at the suture ends are radially stitched through bypass graft and target vessel to complete the anastomosis, whereat in most cases, the coronary wall should be stitched perforating the intima at first. The first two to four stitches may be conducted applying the parachute technique.

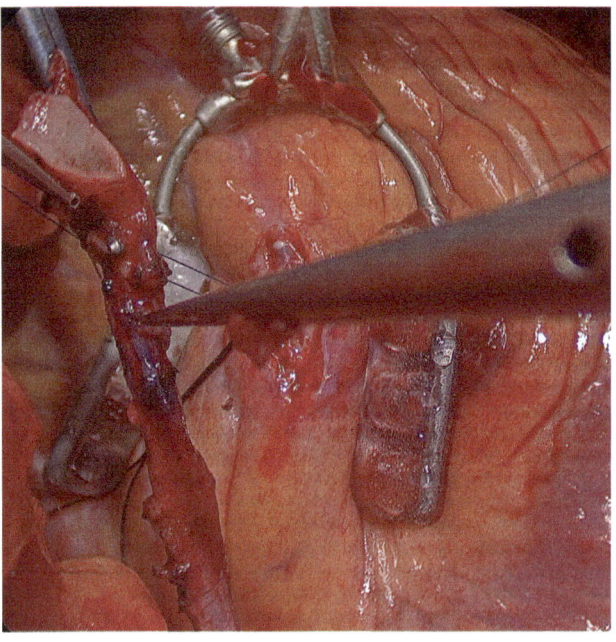

PHOTO 3.65:  Prepared bypass graft

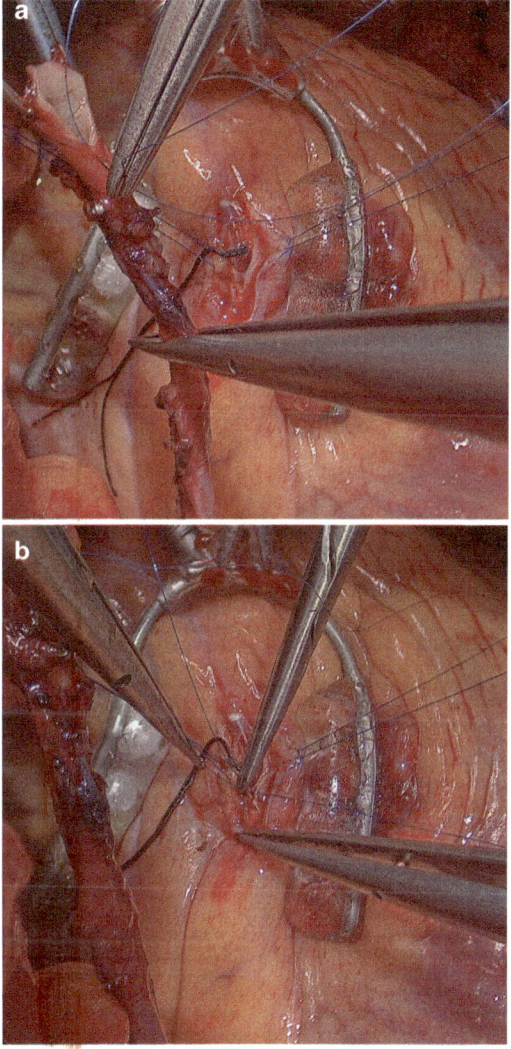

Photo 3.66a+b:  Parachute stitches

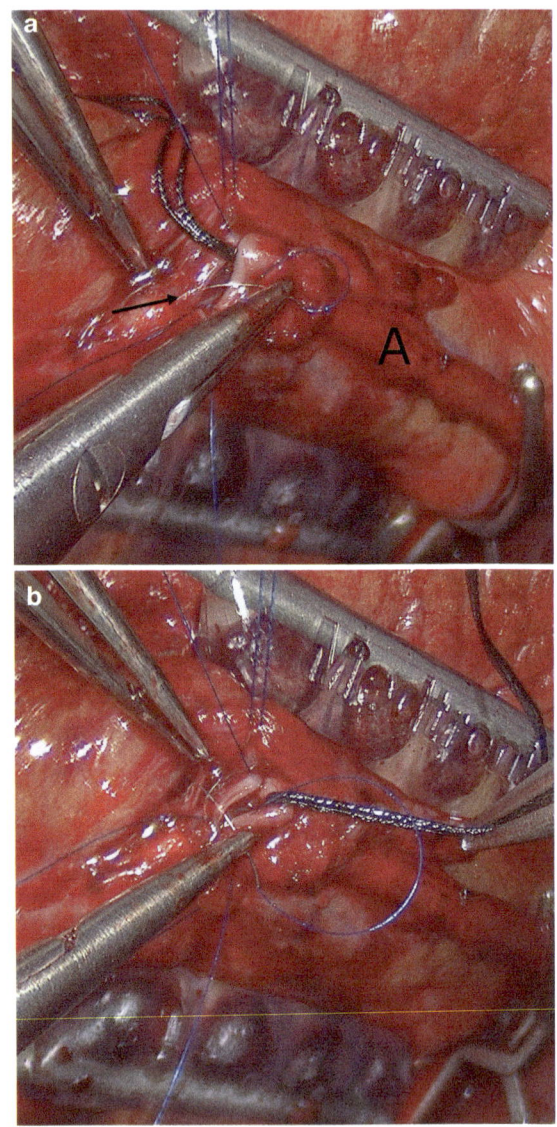

PHOTO 3.67A+B:  a: Toe stitch
→, *toe stitch; A, bypass graft*
b: Toe stitch with shunt support

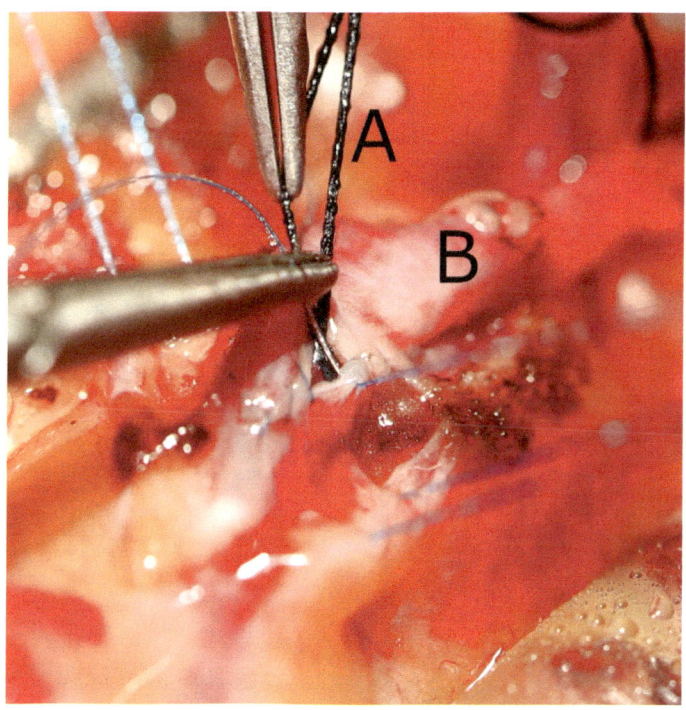

PHOTO 3.68:  Final stitches
*A, shunt support; B, bypass graft*

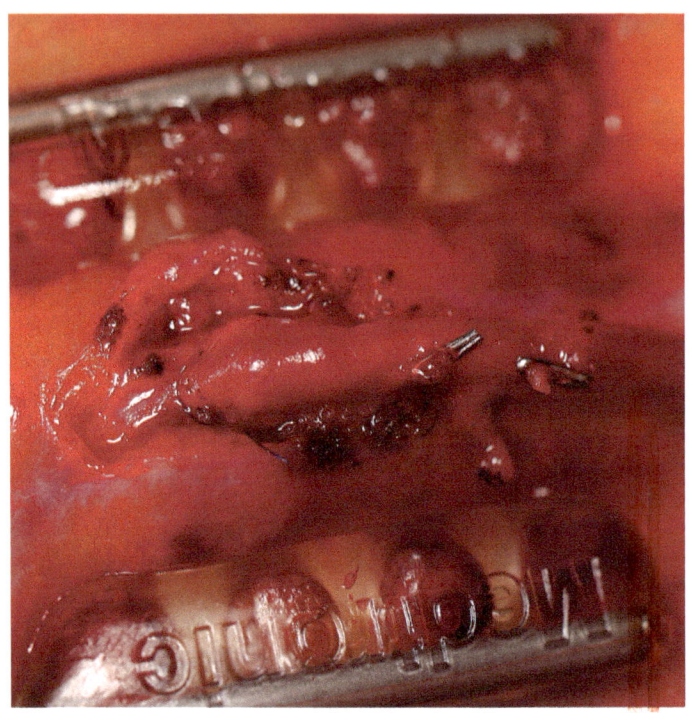

PHOTO 3.69: Completed anastomosis

### 3.5.3.4    Side-to-Side Anastomoses

Side-to-side bypass anastomoses can be sutured in a parallel or an orthogonal fashion, depending on the planned bypass geometry. A common start point of stitching is the area most distant from the surgeon. Starting from there, both needles at the suture ends are radially stitched through bypass graft and target vessel to complete the anastomosis, whereat in most cases, the coronary wall should be stitched perforating the intima at first. The first two to four stitches may be conducted applying the parachute technique.

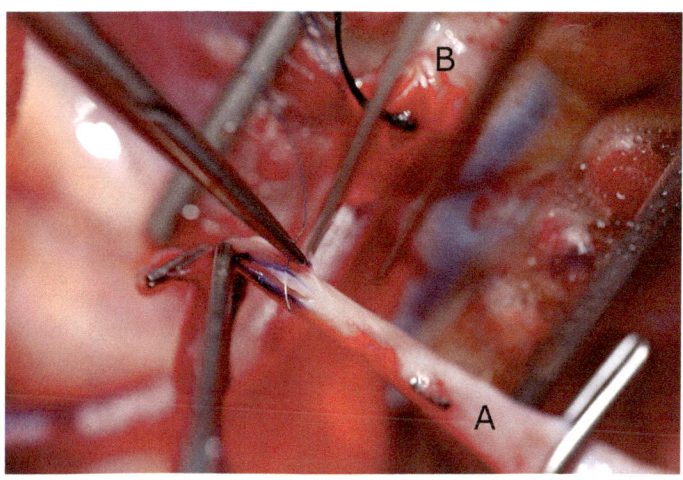

PHOTO 3.70: First stitch
*A, SV; B, native coronary artery with inserted shunt and tissue-everting suture*

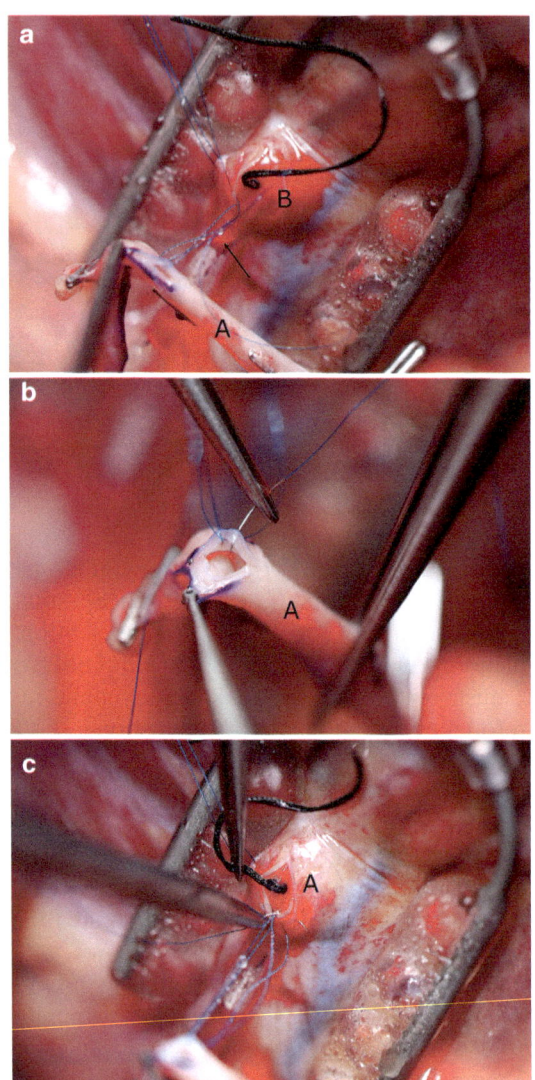

Photo 3.71a–c: a: Parachute stitches
A, SV; B, native coronary artery with inserted shunt and tissue-everting suture, →, parachute stitches
b: Parachute stitches
*A, SV*
c: Parachute stitches
*A, stitch at the native coronary artery with inserted shunt*

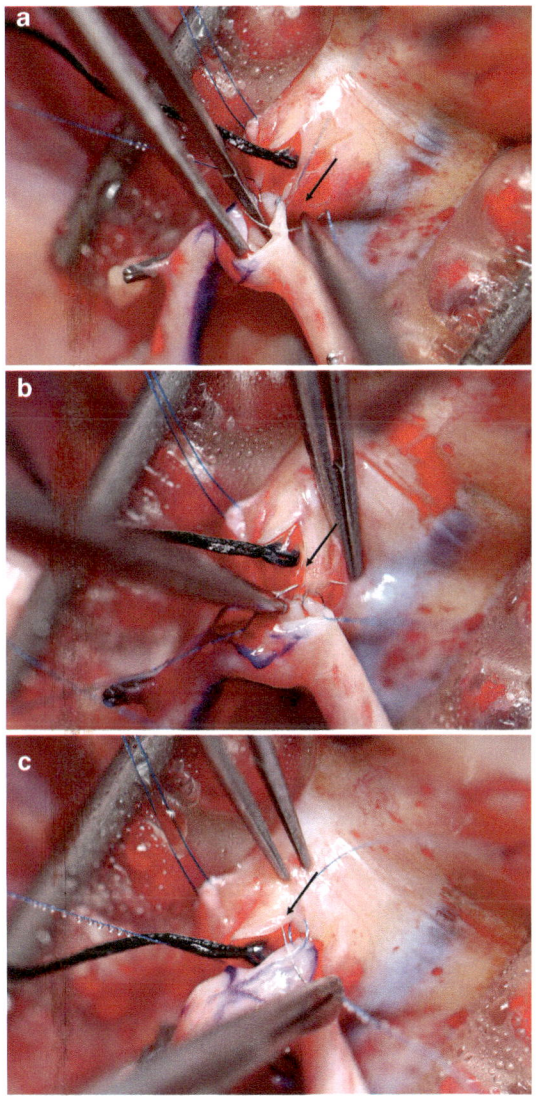

PHOTO 3.72A–C: Surrounding stitches
→, *surrounding stitch*

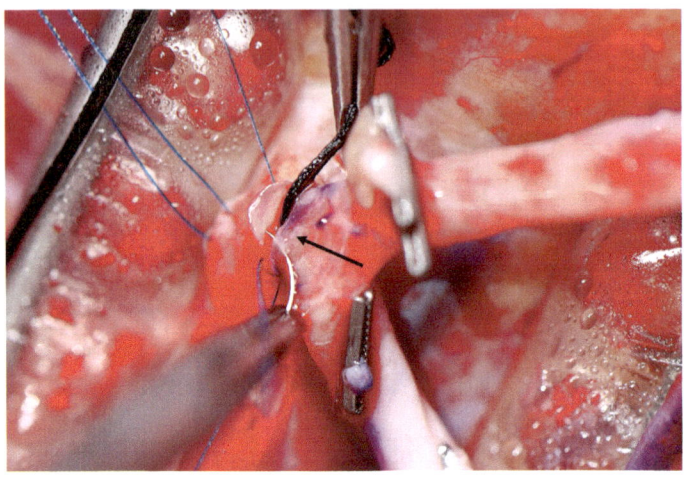

PHOTO 3.73: Final stitches
→, *final stitches with shunt support*

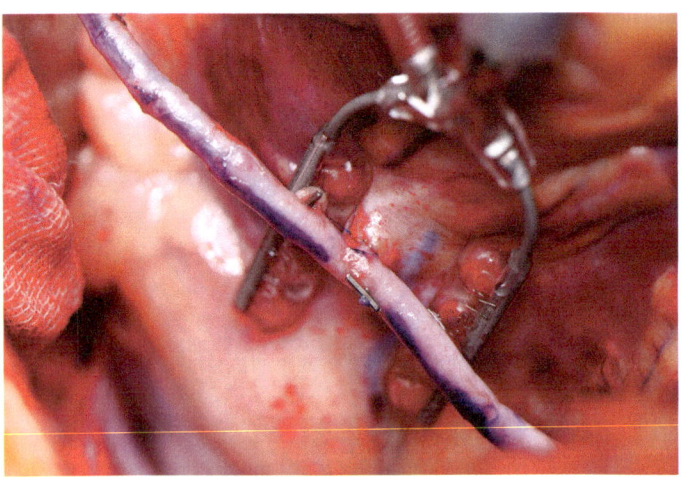

PHOTO 3.74: Completed anastomosis

## 3.6    Flow Measurement

Flow measurement after release of bypass perfusion should be considered to be mandatory to control the patency of the anastomosis.

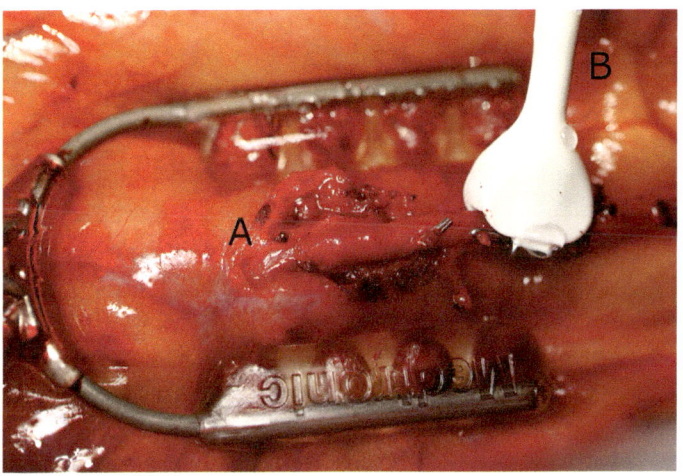

PHOTO 3.75:  Flow measurement
*A, anastomosis; B, flow probe*

## Reference

1. Kawajiri H, Grau JB, Fortier JH, et al. Bilateral internal thoracic artery grafting: in situ or composite? Ann Cardiothorac Surg. 2018;7:673–80.

# Chapter 4
## Prototype Patients

**A. Albert, A. Assmann, and A. K. Assmann**

For many patients, different surgical strategies can be applied to achieve safe and sufficient revascularization. However, the majority of patients can be assigned to a patient prototype whose characteristics clearly favour a dedicated approach (Fig. 4.1). In this chapter, typical patient prototype profiles for the most common operation strategies are presented.

Prototype abbreviations:

BITA        bilateral internal thoracic arteries
CX          left circumflex artery
D           diagonal branch
IM          intermediate artery
LAD         left artery descending
LITA        left internal thoracic artery

———
A. Albert (✉)
Clinic of Dortmund gGmbH - Clinic for Heart Surgery, Beurhausstraße, Germany
e-mail: alexander.albert@klinikumdo.de

A. Assmann · A. K. Assmann
Department of Cardiac Surgery, University Hospital Düsseldorf, Düsseldorf, Nordrhein-Westfalen, Germany
e-mail: alexander.assmann@med.uni-duesseldorf.de;
annakathrin.assmann@med.uni-duesseldorf.de

© Springer Nature Switzerland AG 2021                    113
A. Albert et al. (eds.), *Operative Techniques in Coronary Artery Bypass Surgery*,
https://doi.org/10.1007/978-3-030-48497-2_4

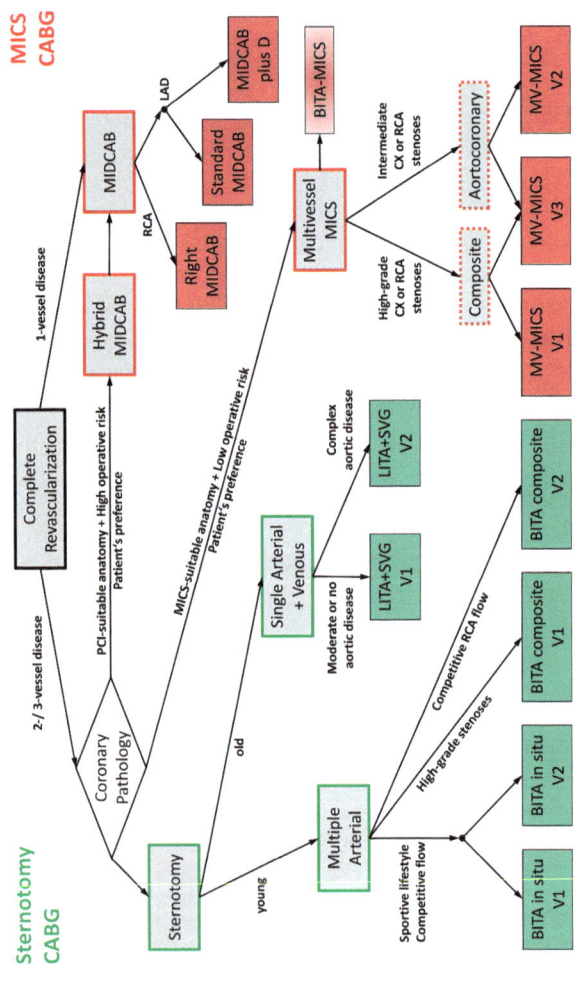

FIGURE 4.1  Decision tree for the CABG strategy. Grey rectangles with coloured frames display operative concepts. Colour-filled rectangles display the MICS CABG (red) and sternotomy CABG (green) prototypes that are presented in detail in the following chapters

| LPL | left posterolateral |
| MV | multivessel |
| OM | obtuse (left) marginal branch |
| PDA | posterior descending artery |
| RA | radial artery |
| RCA | right coronary artery |
| RITA | right internal thoracic artery |
| RPL | right posterolateral branch |
| SV | saphenous vein |
| (xy-)VD | (xy-)vessel coronary artery disease |

Regarding the following prototype profiles, the Syntax score can be calculated to assess the complexity of coronary disease, and the STS score to assess the operative risk.

## 4.1    Left Anterolateral MIDCAB

**Standard:**

1. LITA (*in situ*) → LAD (=Standard MIDCAB)

**Variations:**

1. LITA (*in situ*) → LAD + RA/SV (composite) → D (=MIDCAB plus D)
2. SV (aortic) → CX

### 4.1.1    Standard MIDCAB

LITA (*in situ*) → LAD

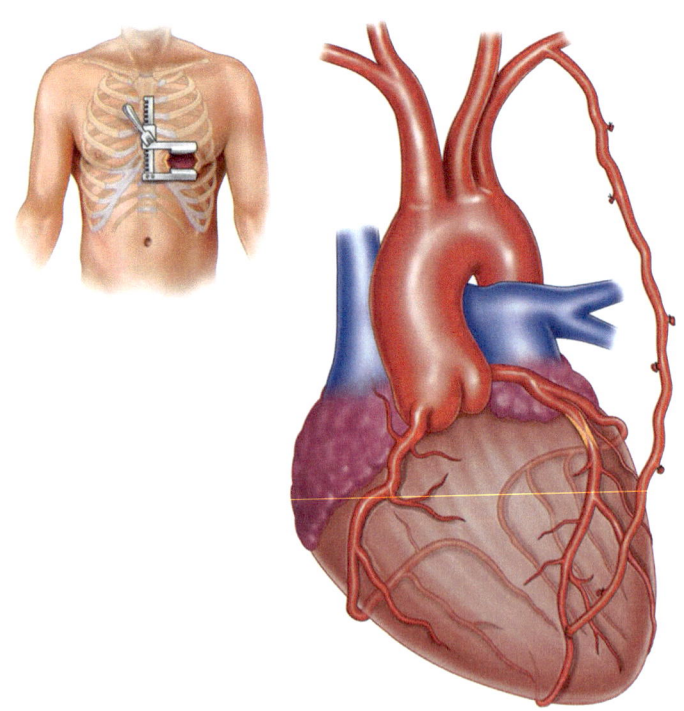

## 4.1.1.1 Prototype Profile

Possible for every patient with single vessel disease of the LAD or as a hybrid procedure.

| | |
|---|---|
| Age | Young → old |
| Coronary pathology | 1-vessel disease (LAD) |
| Residual coronary flow | Low → intermediate |
| Complexity of coronary disease | Low → high |
| Urgency | Elective → urgent |
| Operative risk | Low → high |
| Left ventricular function | Normal → low |
| Aortic atherosclerosis | None → complex |
| Co-morbidities | Sufficient lung function |
| Further aspects | Patient prefers MICS |
| Bypass material | LITA |

Besides standard MIDCAB in coronary 1-vessel disease, multivessel disease patients with high-grade LAD stenosis may be eligible for hybrid approaches, such as in case of poor left ventricular ejection function and complex comorbidities, or in case of emergency non-LAD PCI due to acute ischemia without LAD revascularization.

## 4.1.1.2 Prototype Coronary Angiography

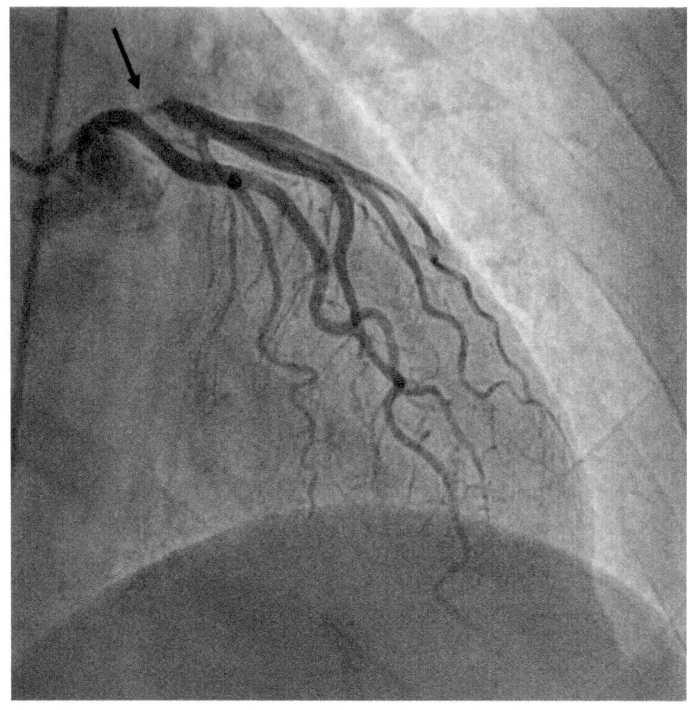

ANGIOGRAM 4.1: Coronary angiogram of the left coronary circulation

→, *LAD stenosis*

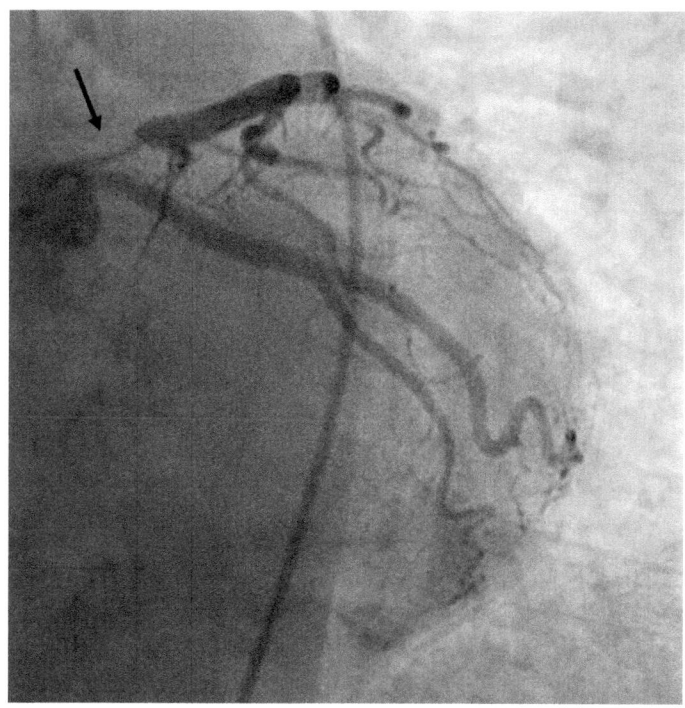

ANGIOGRAM 4.2: Coronary angiogram of the left coronary circulation

→, *LAD stenosis*

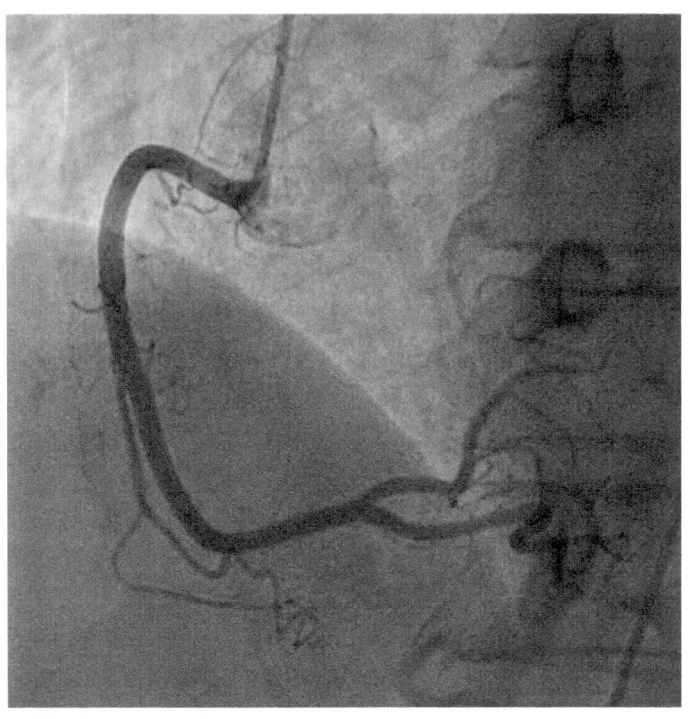

ANGIOGRAM 4.3: Coronary angiogram of the right coronary circulation

## 4.1.1.3   Surgical Technique

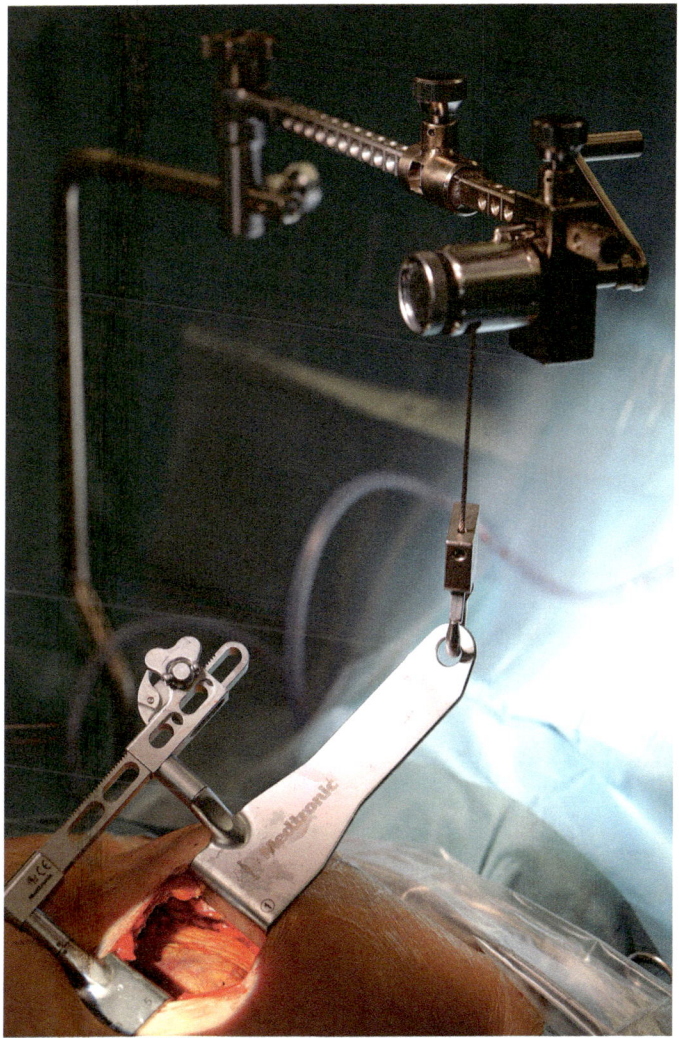

PHOTO 4.1:  MICS retractor installation

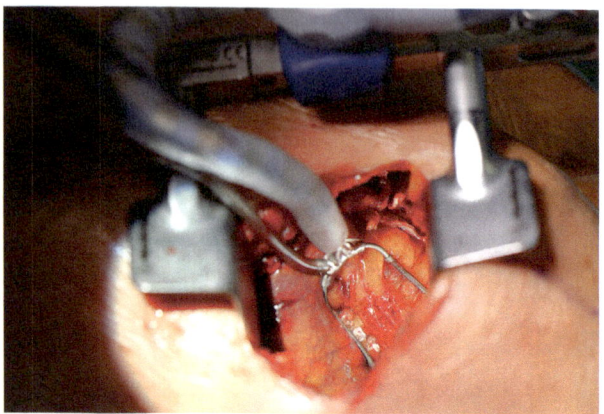

Photo 4.2: MIDCAB installation

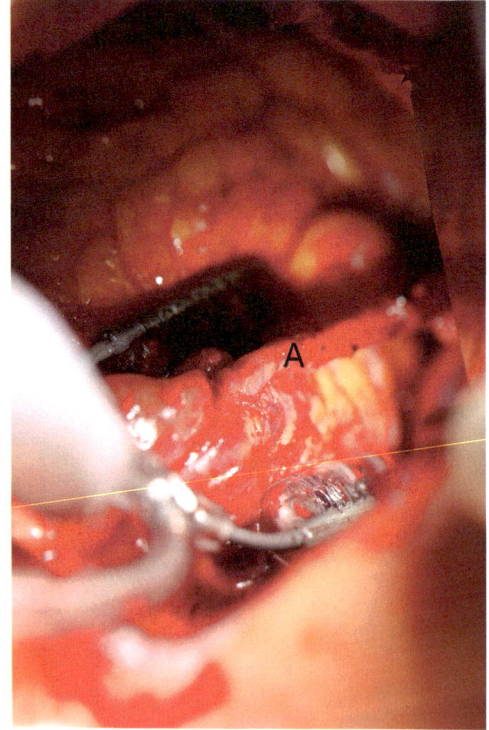

Photo 4.3: LITA (A) to LAD

## 4.1.2   MIDCAB Plus D

LITA (*in situ*) → LAD + RA/SV (composite) → D

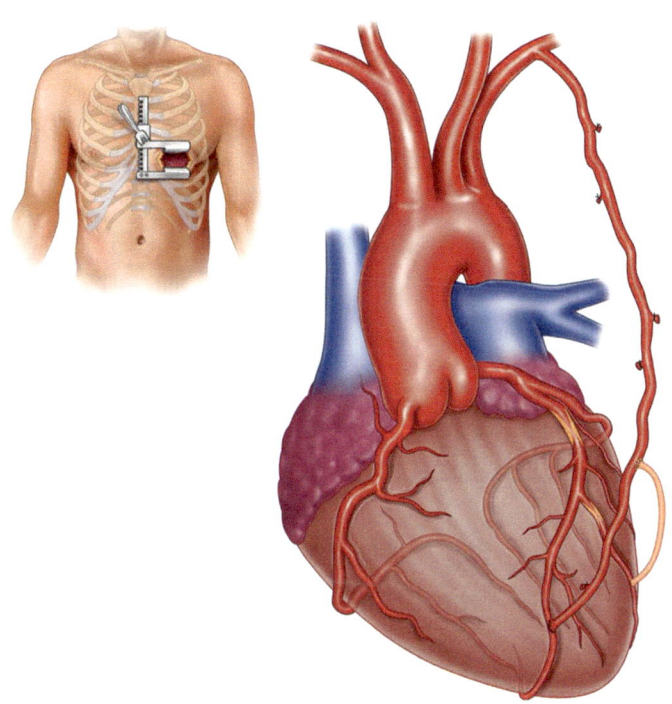

### 4.1.2.1    Prototype Profile

Extended MIDCAB for complete revascularization of the anterior wall.

| | |
|---|---|
| Age | Young → old |
| Coronary pathology | 1-vessel disease (LAD+D) |
| Residual coronary flow | Low → intermediate |
| Complexity of coronary disease | Low → high |
| Urgency | Elective → urgent |
| Operative risk | Low → medium |
| Left ventricular function | Normal → intermediate |
| Aortic atherosclerosis | None → complex |
| Co-morbidities | Sufficient lung function |
| Further aspects | Patient prefers MICS |
| Bypass material | LITA and RA/SV |

## 4.1.2.2   Prototype Coronary Angiography

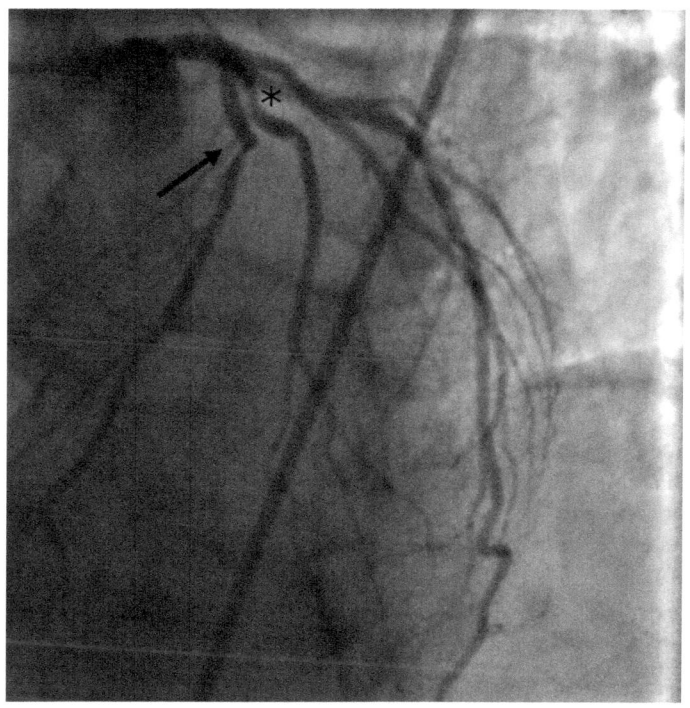

ANGIOGRAM 4.4: Coronary angiogram of the left coronary circulation

→, *LAD stenosis; *, D stenosis*

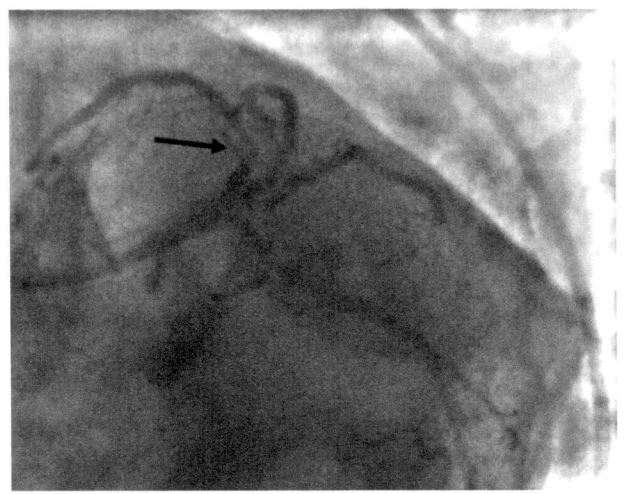

ANGIOGRAM 4.5: Coronary angiogram of the left coronary circulation
→, *LAD stenosis*

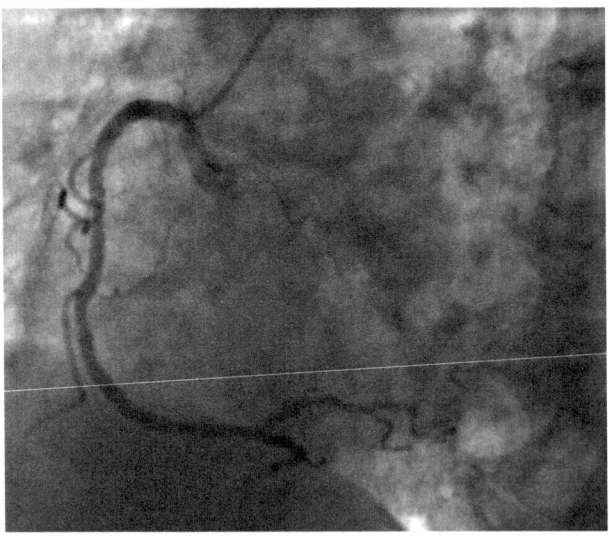

ANGIOGRAM 4.6: Coronary angiogram of the right coronary circulation

## 4.1.2.3   Surgical Technique

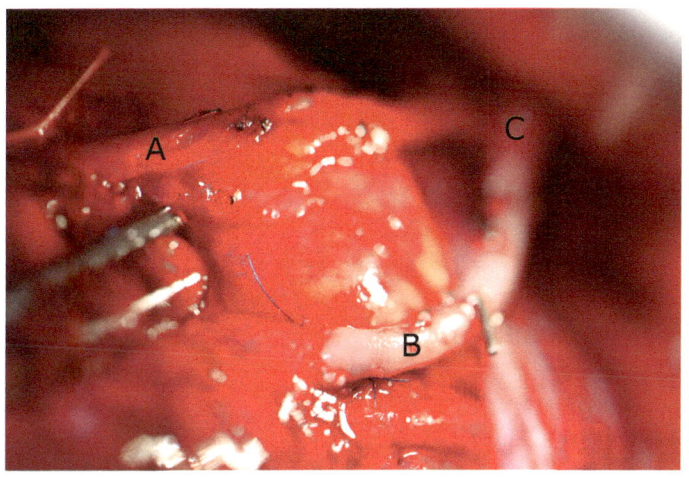

PHOTO 4.4:  LITA to LAD, RA as T-graft to D
*A, LITA to LAD; B, RA to D; C, T-graft*

## 4.2    Right Anterolateral MIDCAB

**Standard:**

1.  SV (aortic) → RCA (=Standard right MIDCAB)

**Variation:**

1.  RITA (*in situ*) → RCA

### *4.2.1    Standard Right MIDCAB*

SV (aortic) → RCA

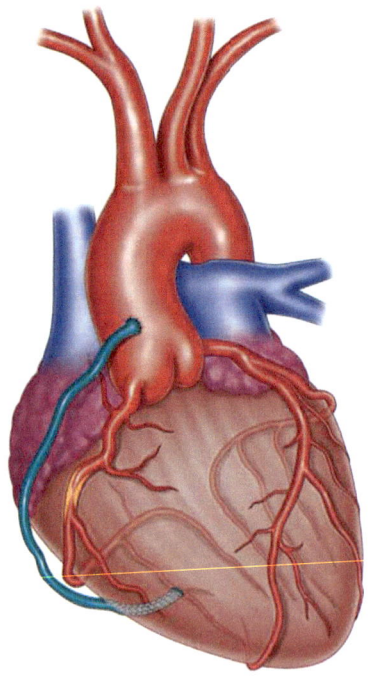
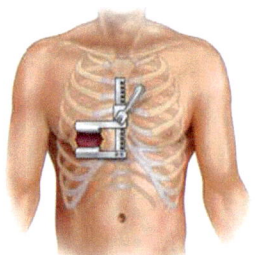

## 4.2.1.1   Prototype Profile

MICS revascularization for clinically significant RCA stenoses (severely diseased vessels or after failed PCI).

| | |
|---|---|
| Age | Young → old |
| Coronary pathology | 1-vessel disease (RCA) |
| Residual coronary flow | Low → intermediate |
| Complexity of coronary disease | Low → intermediate (peripheral RCA or proximal PDA eligible for anastomosis) |
| Urgency | Elective |
| Operative risk | Low → intermediate |
| Left ventricular function | Normal → intermediate |
| Aortic atherosclerosis | None → moderate |
| Co-morbidities | Sufficient lung function |
| Further aspects | Patient prefers MICS |
| Bypass material | SV |

## 4.2.1.2    Prototype Coronary Angiography

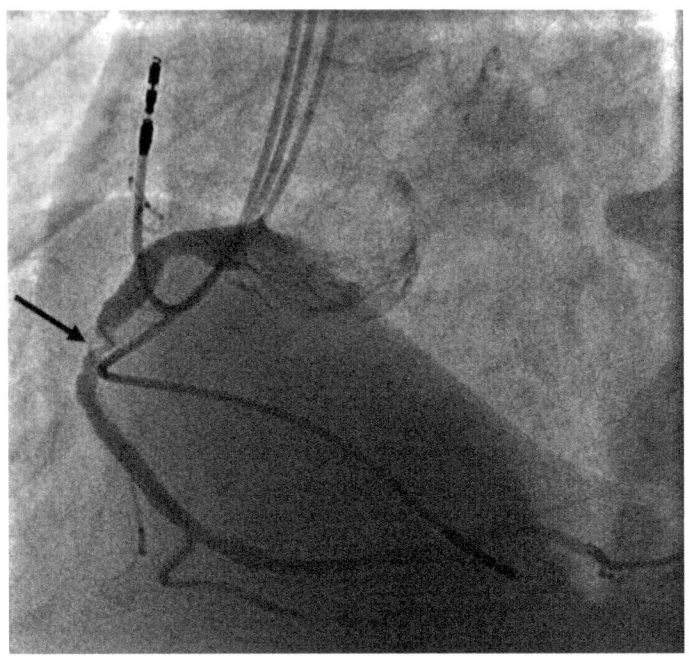

ANGIOGRAM 4.7: Coronary angiogram of the right coronary circulation
→, *RCA stenosis*

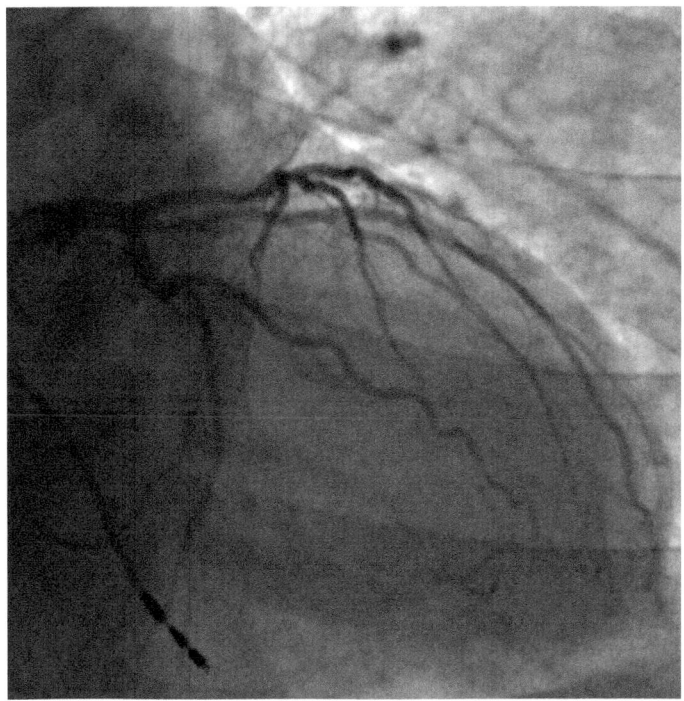

ANGIOGRAM 4.8:  Coronary angiogram of the left coronary circulation

### 4.2.1.3    Surgical Technique

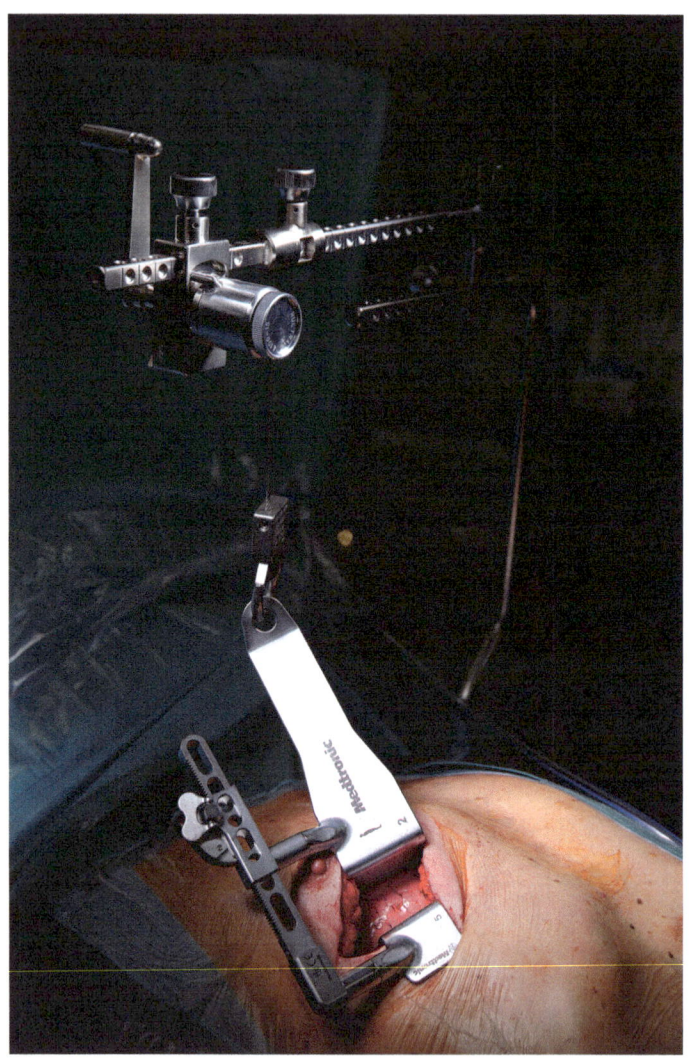

Photo 4.5: Right-sided MICS retractor installation

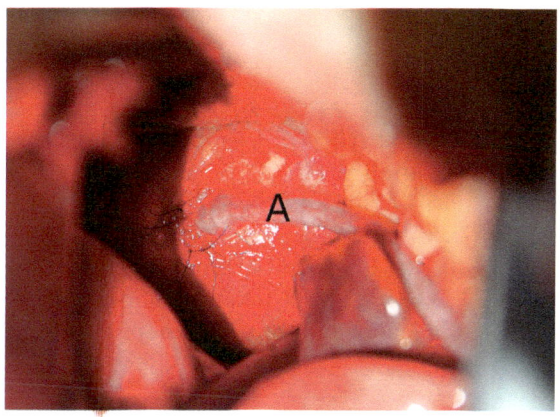

PHOTO 4.6:  Aortic SV to PDA
*A, proximal anastomosis*

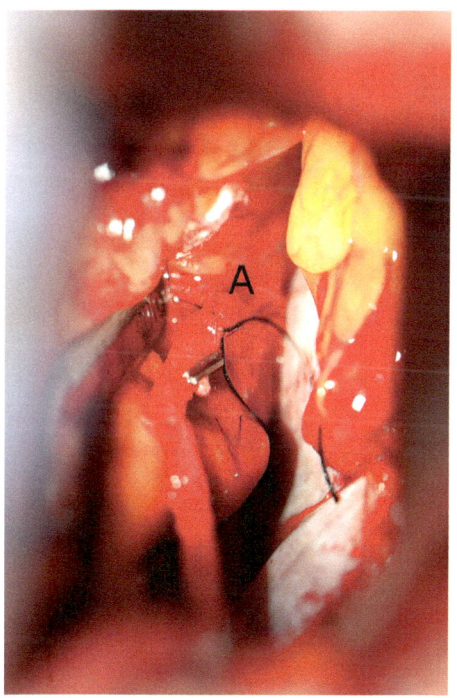

PHOTO 4.7:  Distal anastomosis – SVG to PDA
*A, SVG to PDA*

## 4.3    Multivessel(MV)-MICS

**Variations:**

1. LITA (*in situ*) → LAD + RA (composite) → OM ±PDA (=MV-MICS Variation 1)
2. LITA (*in situ*) → LAD + RA/SV (aortic) → OM ±PDA (=MV-MICS Variation 2)
3. LITA (*in situ*) → LAD + RA (composite) → OM + SV (aortic) → PDA (=MV-MICS Variation 3)
4. BITA-MICS: Please see a separate chapter following this prototype chapter

### *4.3.1    MV-MICS Variation 1*

LITA (*in situ*) → LAD + RA (composite) → OM ±PDA

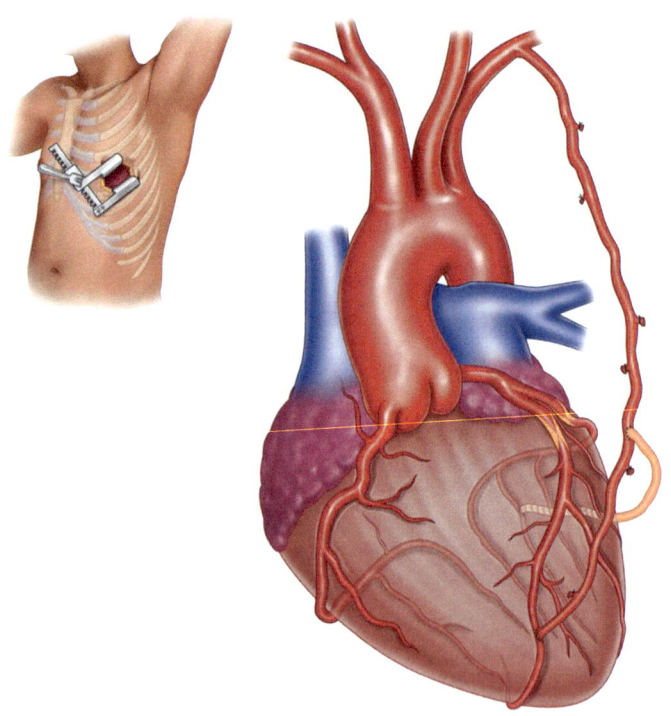

## 4.3.1.1   Prototype Profile

MICS multivessel procedure in the presence of high-grade CX or RCA stenosis, respectively.

| Age | Young |
|---|---|
| Coronary pathology | 2-/3-vessel disease (LAD+CX±RCA), high-grade stenoses in CX/RCA |
| Residual coronary flow | Low (LAD+CX±RCA) → intermediate (LAD) |
| Complexity of coronary disease | Low → intermediate |
| Urgency | Elective |
| Operative risk | Low |
| Left ventricular function | Normal → intermediate |
| Aortic atherosclerosis | None ("anaortic OPCAB" possible) |
| Co-morbidities | Sufficient lung function, no history of stroke, no generalized atherosclerosis, adequate body shape, cardio-thoracic ratio <0.5, left ventricular end-diastolic diameter <55 mm |
| Further aspects | Patient explicitly prefers MICS |
| Bypass material | LITA and RA |

## 4.3.1.2    Prototype Coronary Angiography

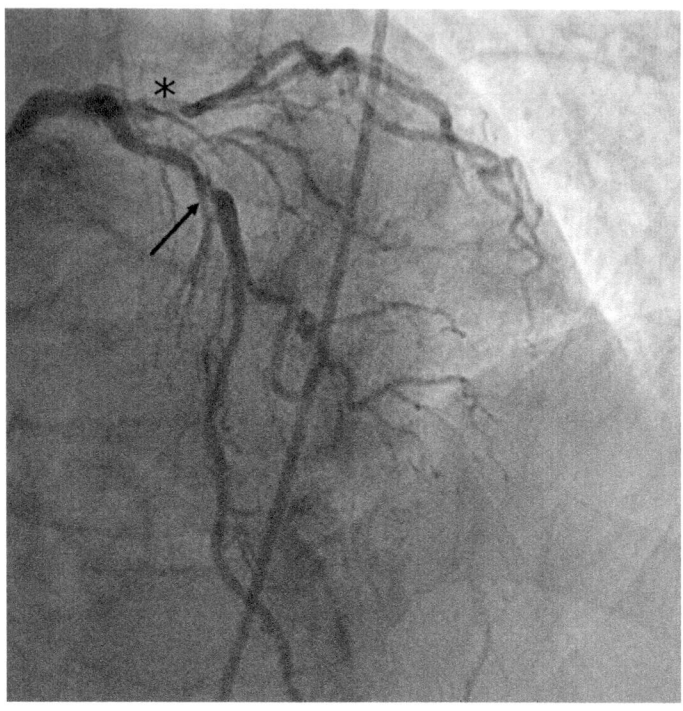

ANGIOGRAM 4.9: Coronary angiogram of the left coronary circulation
→, *LAD stenosis; *, CX stenosis*

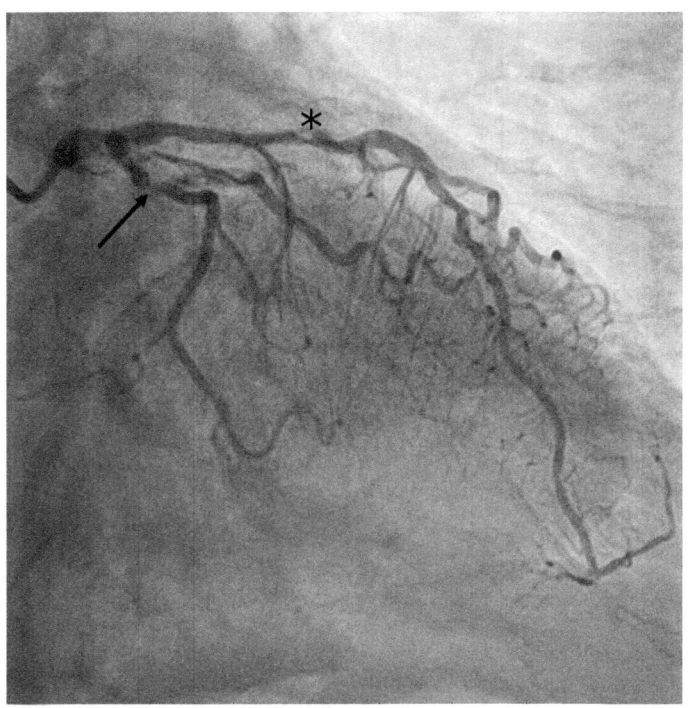

ANGIOGRAM 4.10: Coronary angiogram of the left coronary circulation

→, *CX stenosis; * LAD stenosis*

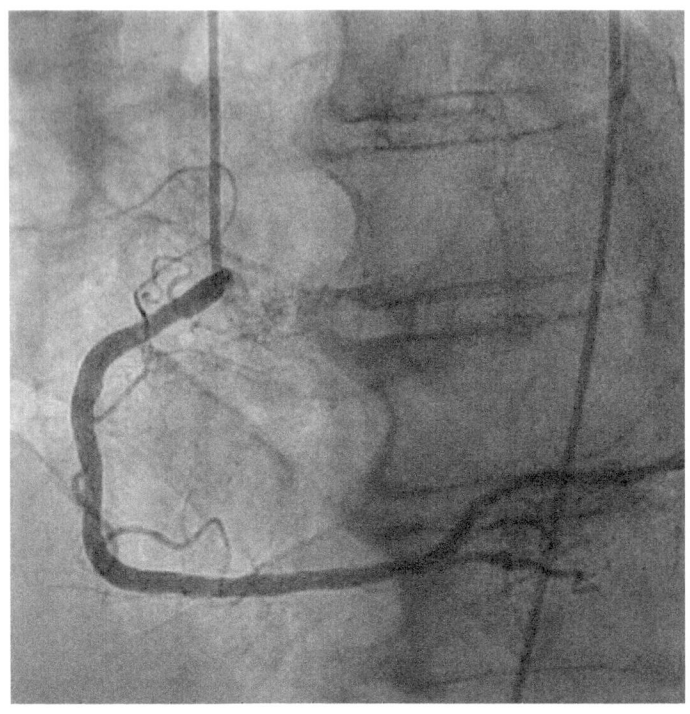

ANGIOGRAM 4.11: Coronary angiogram of the right coronary circulation

## 4.3.1.3   Surgical Technique

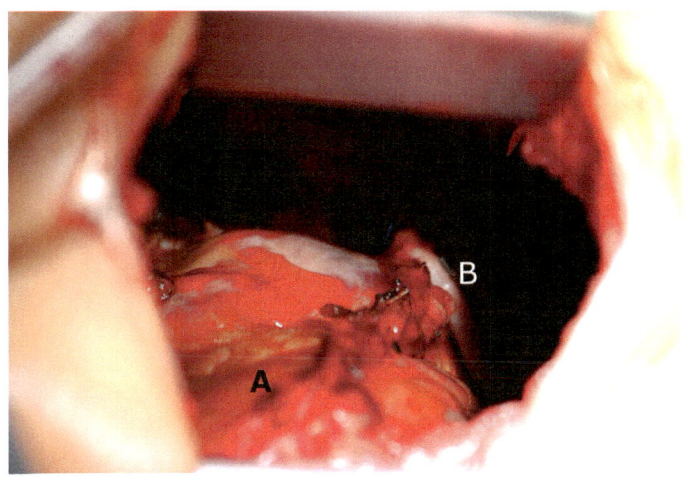

Photo 4.8:  LITA to LAD and RA to OM
*A, LITA to LAD; B, RA T-graft from LITA*

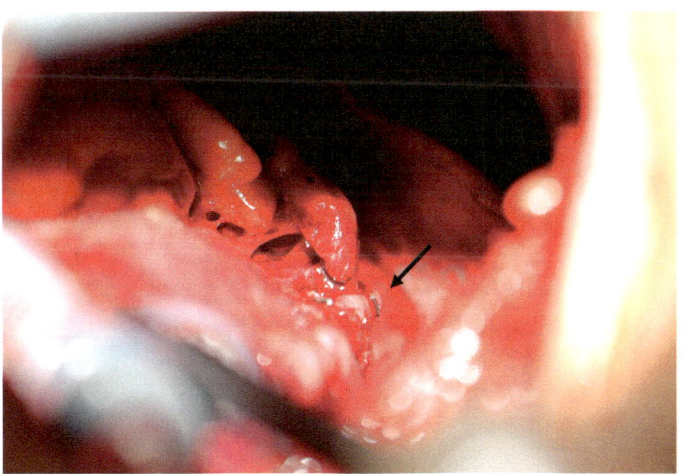

Photo 4.9:  Distal anastomosis
→, *RA to OM*

### 4.3.2    MV-MICS Variation 2

LITA (*in situ*) → LAD + RA/SV (aortic) → OM ±PDA

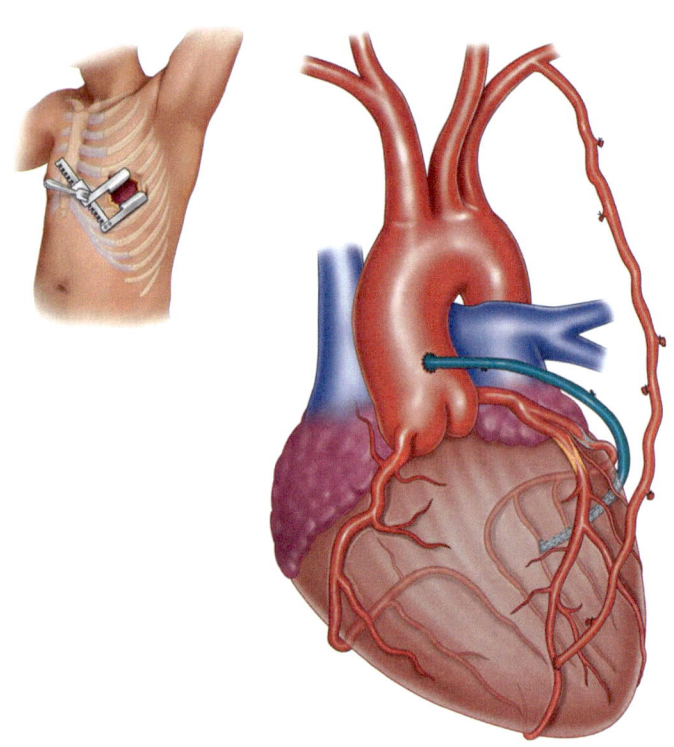

## 4.3.2.1  Prototype Profile

MICS multivessel procedure in the presence of *non*-high-grade CX or RCA stenosis, respectively.

| | |
|---|---|
| Age | Young |
| Coronary pathology | 2-/3-vessel disease (LAD+CX±RCA), intermediate or high-grade stenoses in CX/RCA |
| Residual coronary flow | Low → intermediate |
| Complexity of coronary disease | Low → intermediate |
| Urgency | Elective |
| Operative risk | Low |
| Left ventricular function | Normal → intermediate |
| Aortic atherosclerosis | None ("clampless OPCAB" possible) |
| Co-morbidities | Sufficient lung function, no history of stroke, no generalized atherosclerosis, adequate body shape, cardio-thoracic ratio <0.5, left ventricular end-diastolic diameter <55 mm |
| Further aspects | Patient explicitly prefers MICS |
| Bypass material | LITA and RA/SV |

## 4.3.2.2    Prototype Coronary Angiography

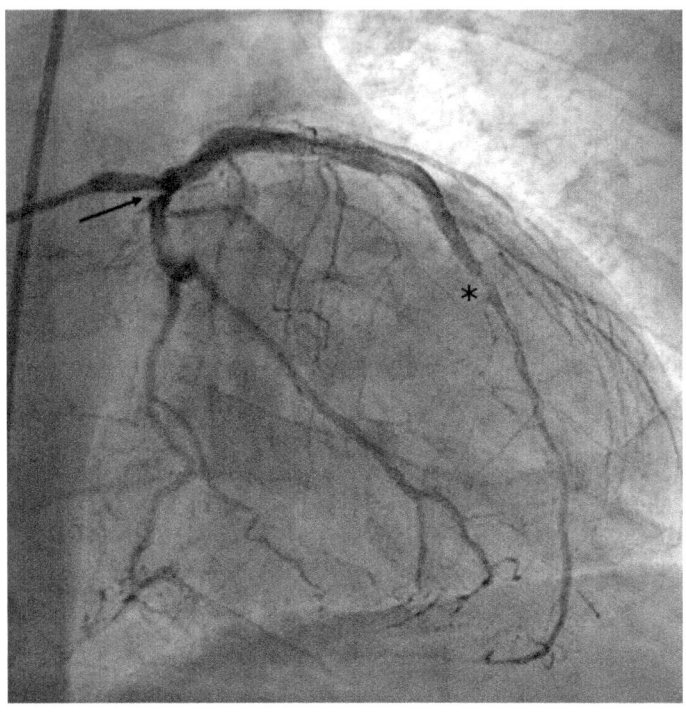

ANGIOGRAM 4.12: Coronary angiogram of the left coronary circulation
→, *left main (LM) stenosis; *, LAD stenosis*

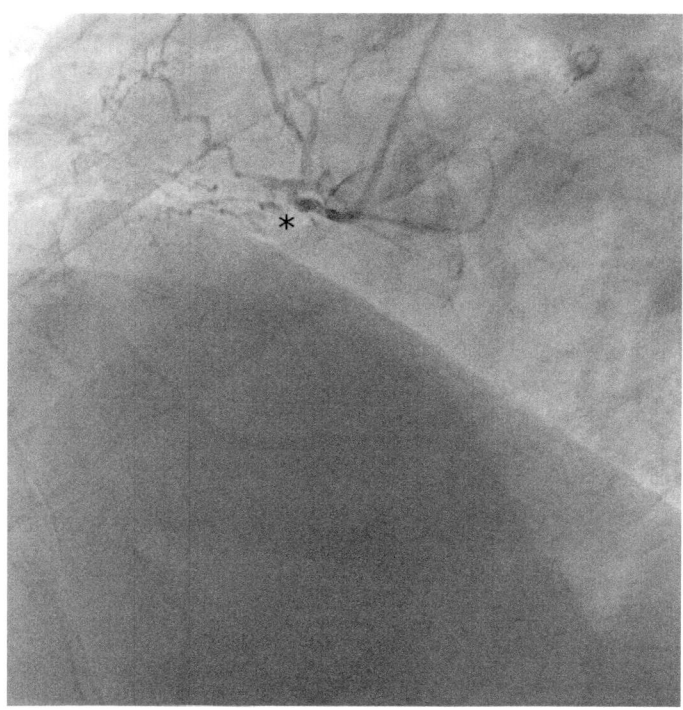

ANGIOGRAM 4.13: Coronary angiogram of the right coronary circulation
*, *RCA chronic total occlusion (CTO)*

## 4.3.2.3   Surgical Technique

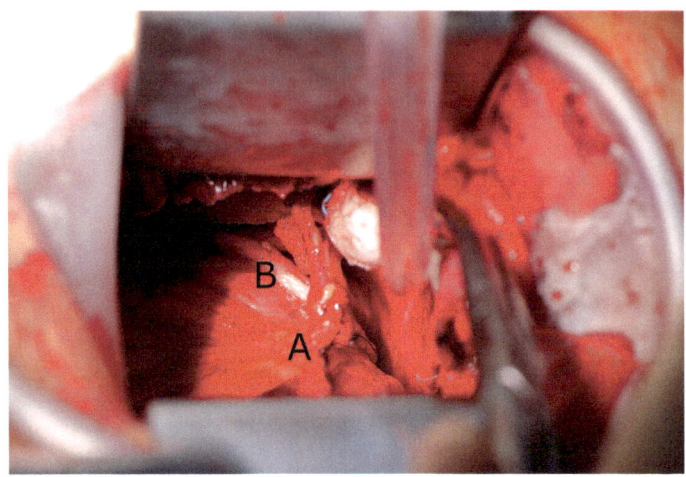

PHOTO 4.10:  LITA to LAD and SV to OM I
*A, LITA TO LAD, B, SV*

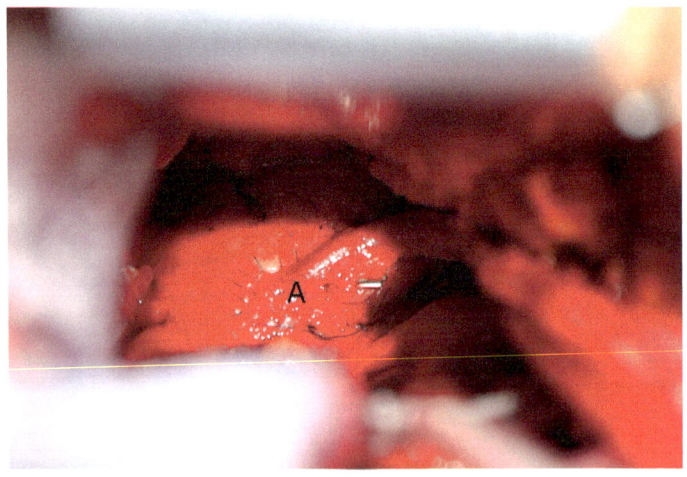

PHOTO 4.11: Aortic anastomosis
*A, aortic anastomosis*

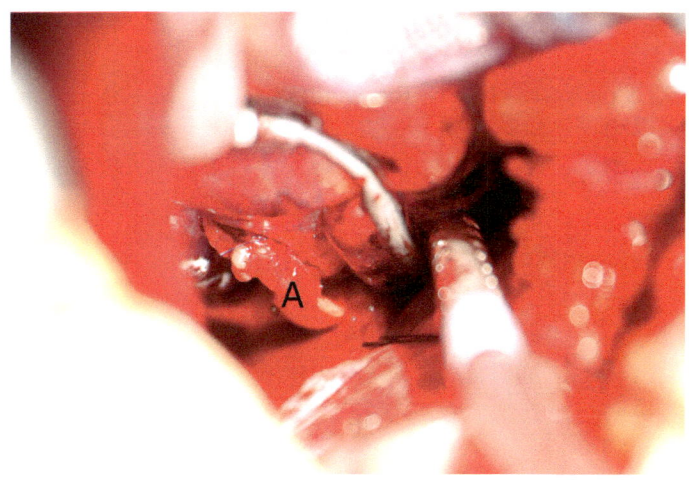

PHOTO 4.12:  Distal anastomosis
*A, SV to OM I*

### 4.3.3    MV-MICS Variation 3

LITA (*in situ*) → LAD + RA (composite) → OM + SV (aortic) → PDA

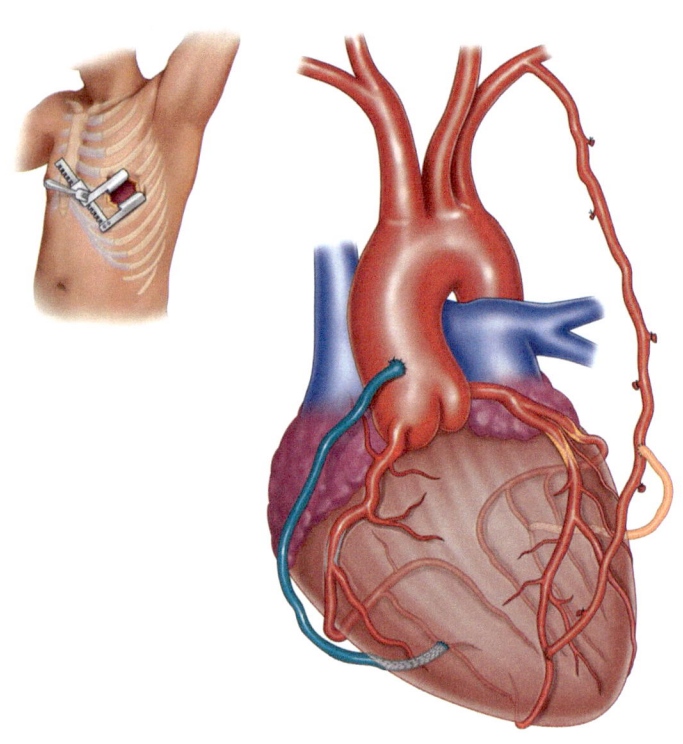

## 4.3.3.1    Prototype Profile

Complex MICS multivessel revascularization for younger patients with explicit wish for MICS.

| Age | Young |
| --- | --- |
| Coronary pathology | 3-vessel disease (LAD+CX+RCA), high-grade stenosis in CX, intermediate or high-grade stenosis in RCA |
| Residual coronary flow | Low (LAD+CX+RCA) → intermediate (LAD+RCA) |
| Complexity of coronary disease | Low → intermediate |
| Urgency | Elective |
| Operative risk | Low |
| Left ventricular function | Normal → intermediate |
| Aortic atherosclerosis | None ("clampless OPCAB" possible) |
| Co-morbidities | Sufficient lung function, no history of stroke, no generalized atherosclerosis, adequate body shape, cardio-thoracic ratio <0.5, left ventricular end-diastolic diameter <55 mm |
| Further aspects | Patient explicitly prefers MICS |
| Bypass material | LITA and RA and SV |

### 4.3.3.2    Prototype Coronary Angiography

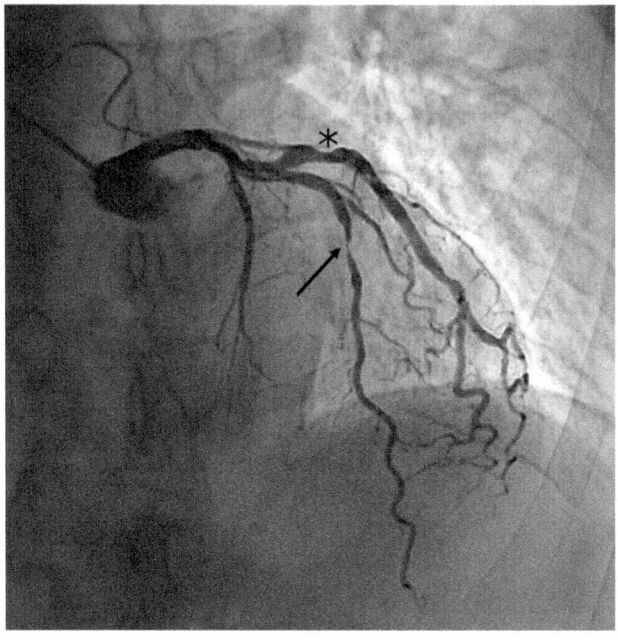

ANGIOGRAM 4.14: Coronary angiogram of the left coronary circulation
→, *LAD stenosis; *, CX stenosis*

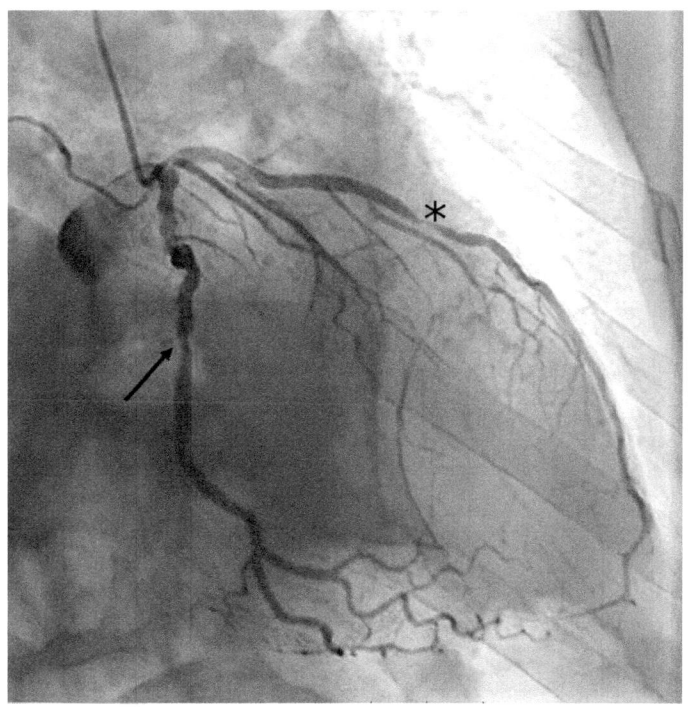

ANGIOGRAM 4.15: Coronary angiogram of the left coronary circulation
→, *CX stenosis; \*, LAD stenosis*

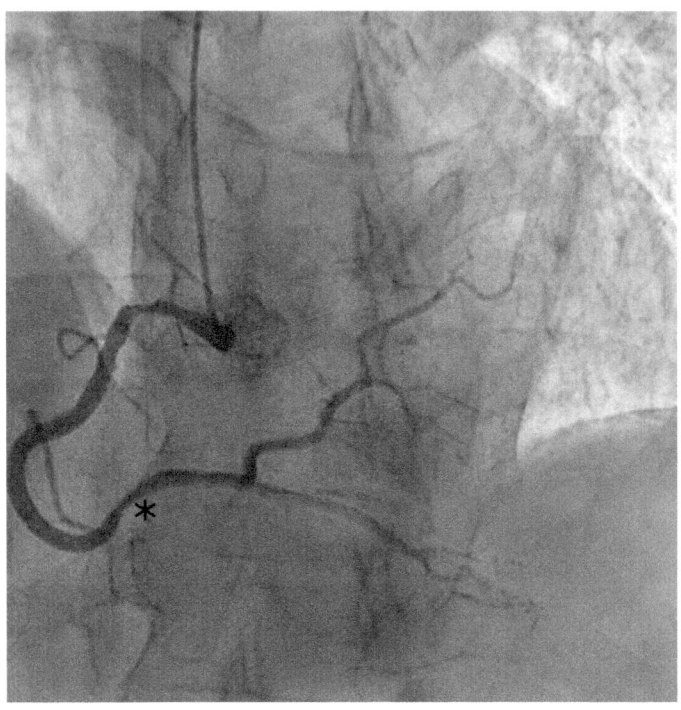

ANGIOGRAM 4.16: Coronary angiogram of the right coronary circulation
*, RCA stenosis

## 4.3.3.3   Surgical Technique

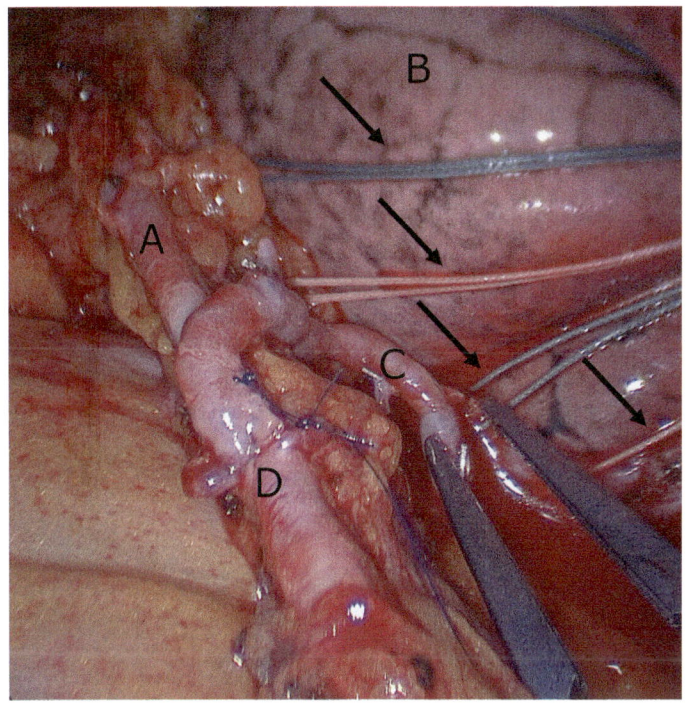

PHOTO 4.13:  LITA to LAD and RA as T-Graft
→, *pulmonary-fan technique for double lung ventilation; A, proximal LITA; B, lung; C, RA; D, T-Graft anastomosis*

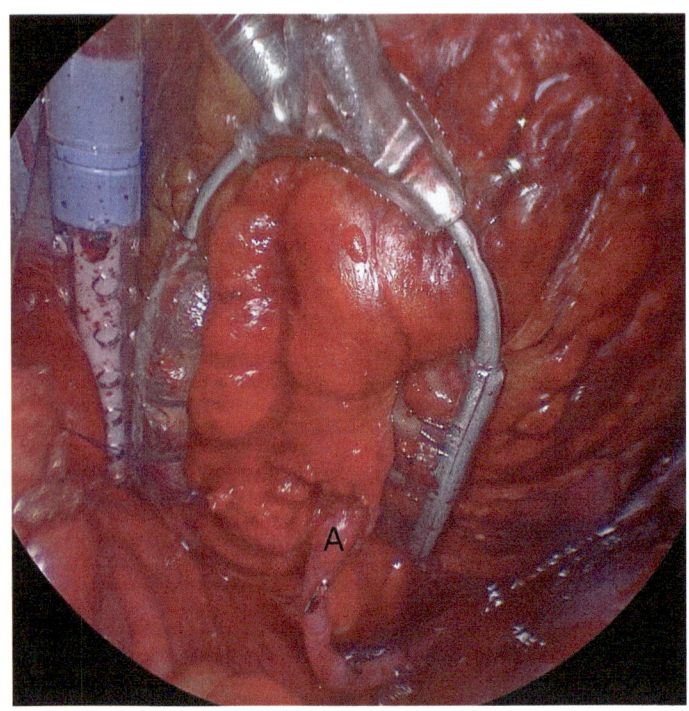

PHOTO 4.14: Distal anastomosis: RA to OM
*A, anastomosis*

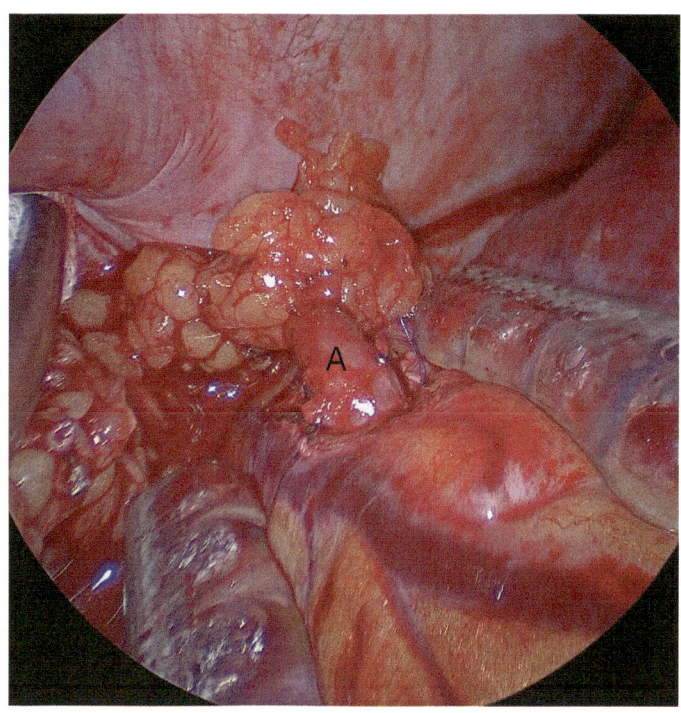

PHOTO 4.15:  Distal anastomosis: SV to PDA
*A, anastomosis*

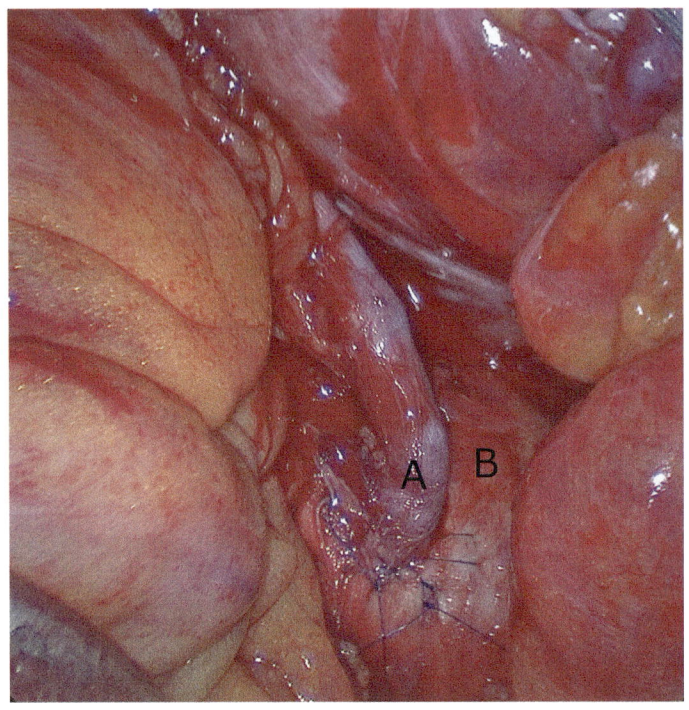

Photo 4.16: Aortic anastomosis
*A, anastomosis; B, aorta*

## 4.4   Multiple Arterial Grafting

**Variations:**

1. BITA (*in situ*) ± RA/SV (aortic) (=BITA *in situ* Variation 1)
2. BITA (*in situ*) + RA elongation for RITA ± RA (aortic) (=BITA *in situ* Variation 2)
3. LITA (*in situ*) + (sequential) RITA (composite) (BITA composite Variation 1)
   Sub-variation: additional mini-T-grafts instead of sequential anastomoses
4. LITA (*in situ*) + RITA (composite) + RA/SV (aortic) (BITA composite Variation 2)


### *4.4.1   BITA In Situ Variation 1*

BITA (*in situ*) ± RA/SV (aortic)

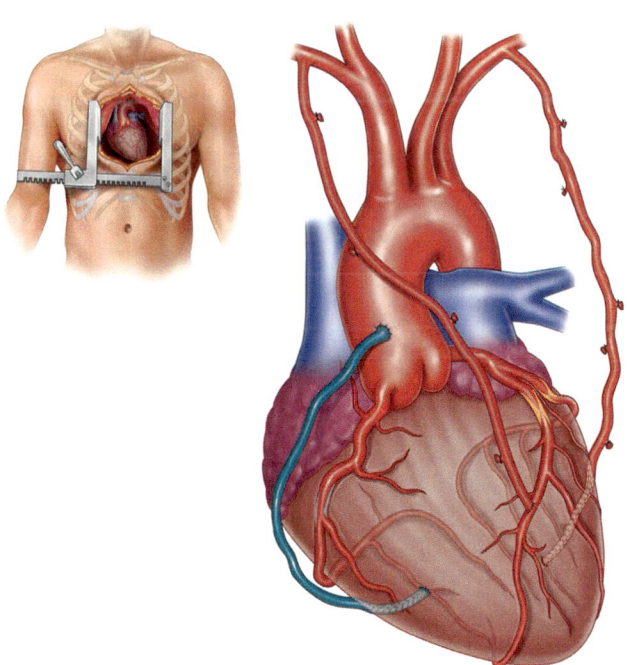

## 4.4.1.1    Prototype Profile

Extended arterial grafting for young patients with sportive lifestyle and risk of competitive RCA flow.

| Age | Young |
|---|---|
| Coronary pathology | 2-/3-vessel disease (LAD+CX±RCA), suitable coronary geometry |
| Residual coronary flow | Low (LAD+CX) → intermediate (LAD+CX±RCA) |
| Complexity of coronary disease | Low → high |
| Urgency | Elective → emergency |
| Operative risk | Low → intermediate |
| Left ventricular function | Normal → intermediate |
| Aortic atherosclerosis | None → moderate ("anaortic or clampless OPCAB") |
| Co-morbidities | Low risk of sternal wound infection |
| Further aspects | Active lifestyle, multiple inflows provide improved perfusion and physical resilience |
| Bypass material | BITA and RA/SV |

## 4.4.1.2    Prototype Coronary Angiography

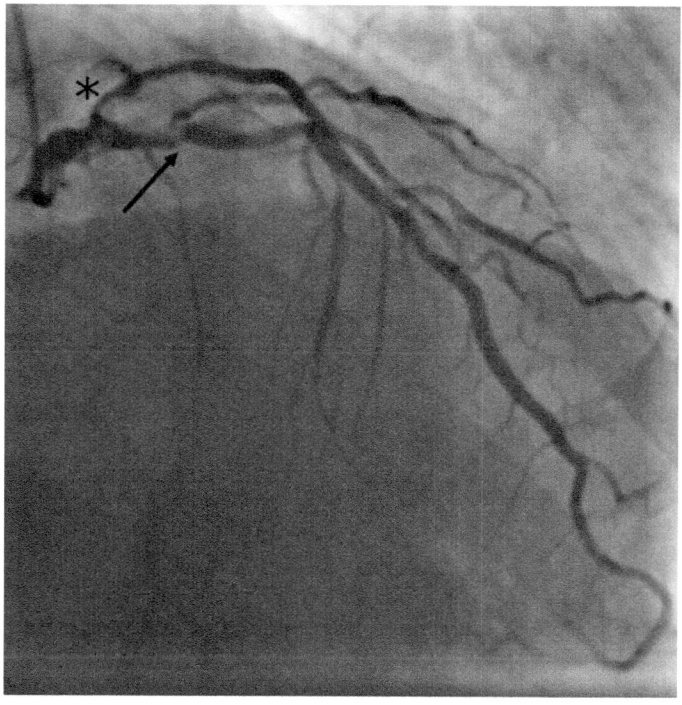

ANGIOGRAM 4.17: Coronary angiogram of the left coronary circulation
→, *LAD stenosis; *, CX stenosis*

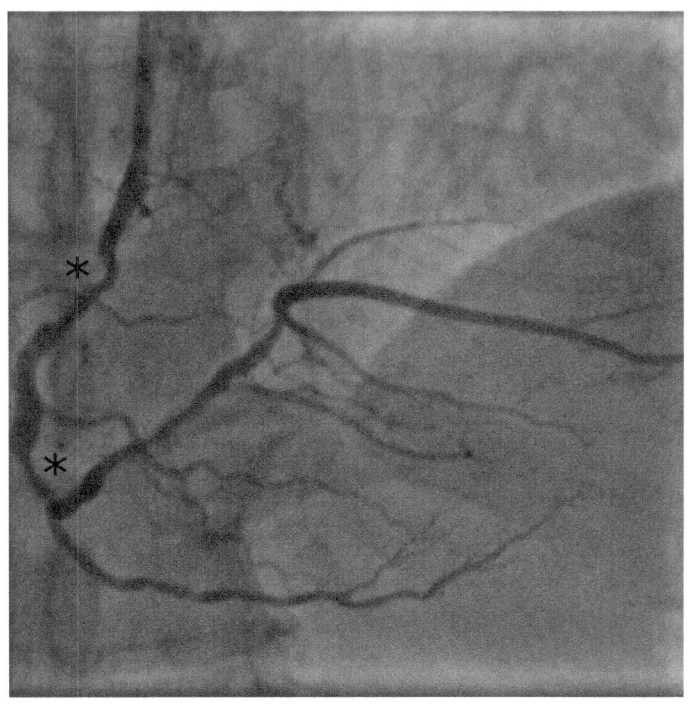

ANGIOGRAM 4.18  Coronary angiogram of the right coronary circulation
*, RCA stenoses

## 4.4.1.3    Surgical Technique

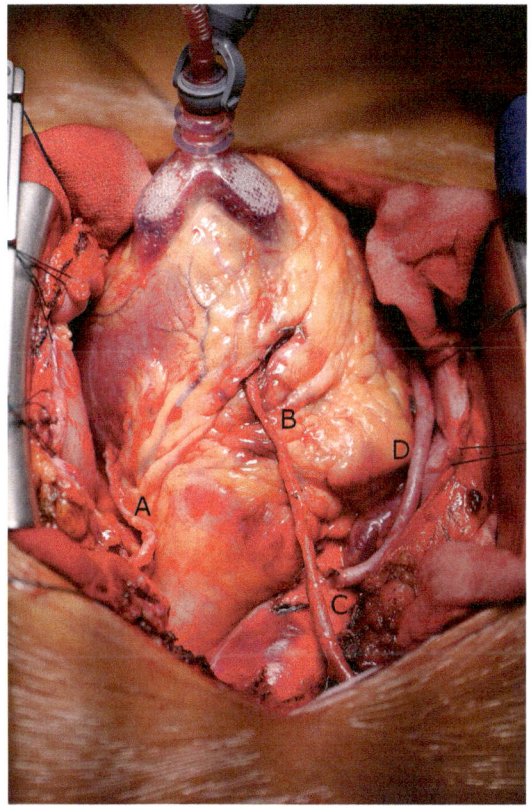

PHOTO 4.17:  RITA to LAD, LITA to OM and SV to RPL
*A, LITA; B, RITA; C, aortic anastomosis; D, SV*

### 4.4.2    BITA In Situ Variation 2

BITA (*in situ*) + RA elongation for RITA ± RA (aortic/ composite)

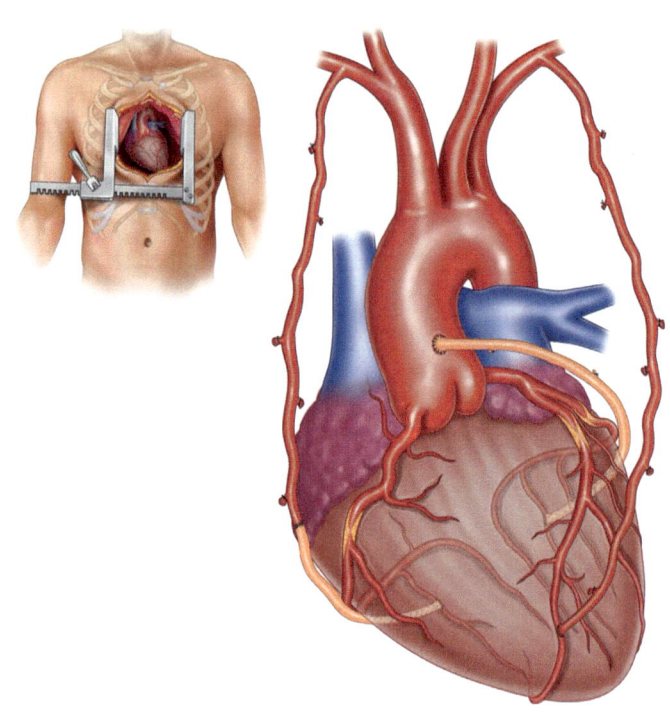

## 4.4.2.1    Prototype Profile

Total arterial grafting with multiple inflows for young patients with sportive lifestyle.

| | |
|---|---|
| Age | Young |
| Coronary pathology | 2-/3-vessel disease (LAD+CX±RCA), suitable coronary geometry |
| Residual coronary flow | Low → intermediate |
| Complexity of coronary disease | Low → high |
| Urgency | Elective → urgent |
| Operative risk | Low → intermediate |
| Left ventricular function | Normal → intermediate |
| Aortic atherosclerosis | None → moderate ("anaortic or clampless OPCAB") |
| Co-morbidities | Low risk of sternal wound infection |
| Further aspects | Active lifestyle, multiple inflows provide improved perfusion and physical resilience |
| Bypass material | BITA and RA |

## 4.4.2.2    Prototype Coronary Angiography

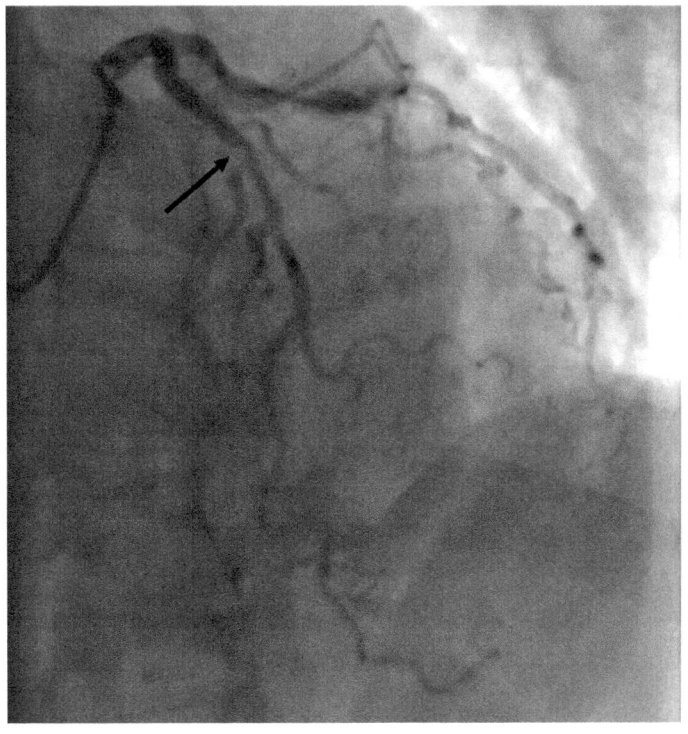

ANGIOGRAM 4.19: Coronary angiogram of the left coronary circulation
→, *LAD stenosis*

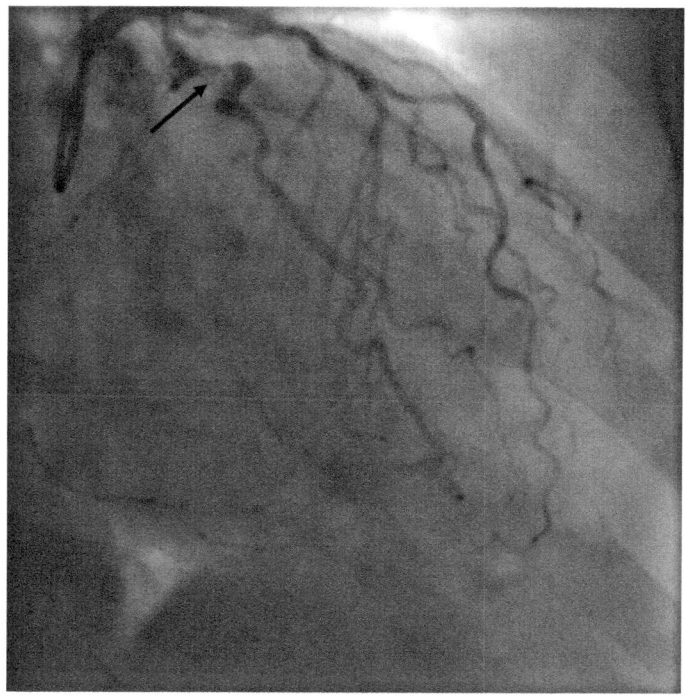

ANGIOGRAM 4.20: Coronary angiogram of the left coronary circulation

→, *CX stenosis*

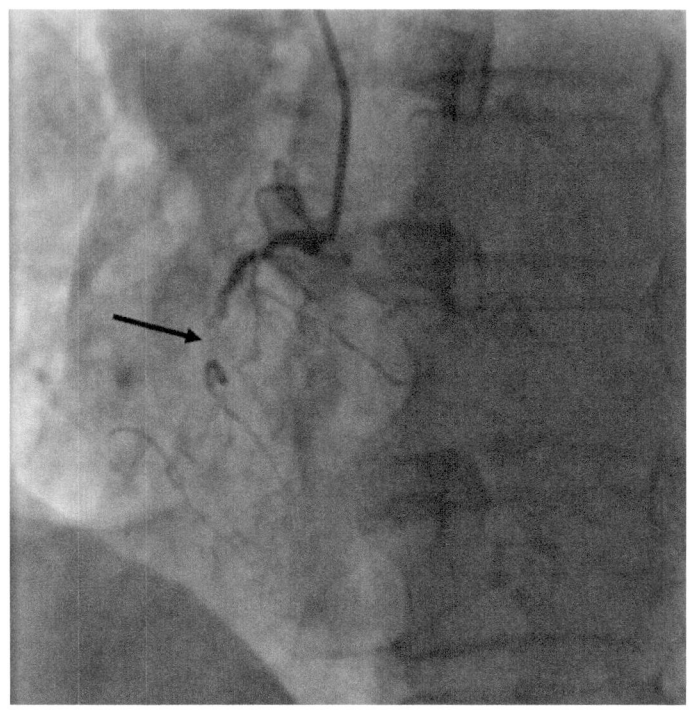

ANGIOGRAM 4.21: Coronary angiogram of the right coronary circulation
→, *RCA CTO*

## 4.4.2.3   Surgical Technique

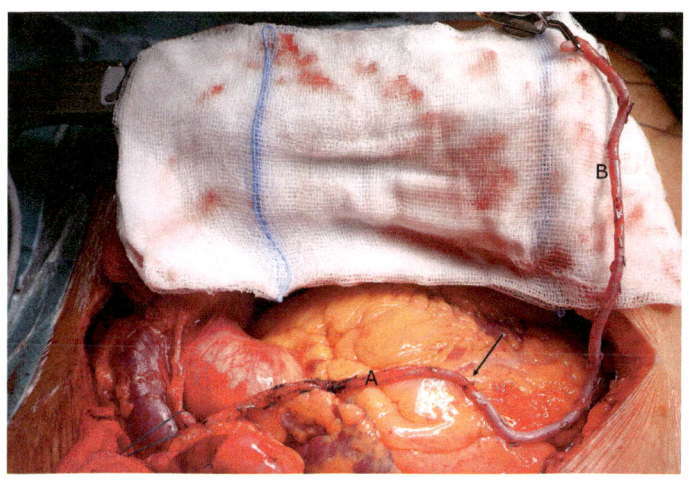

Photo 4.18:  Radial artery elongation for RITA
→ *end-to-end anastomosis; A, RITA; B, RA*

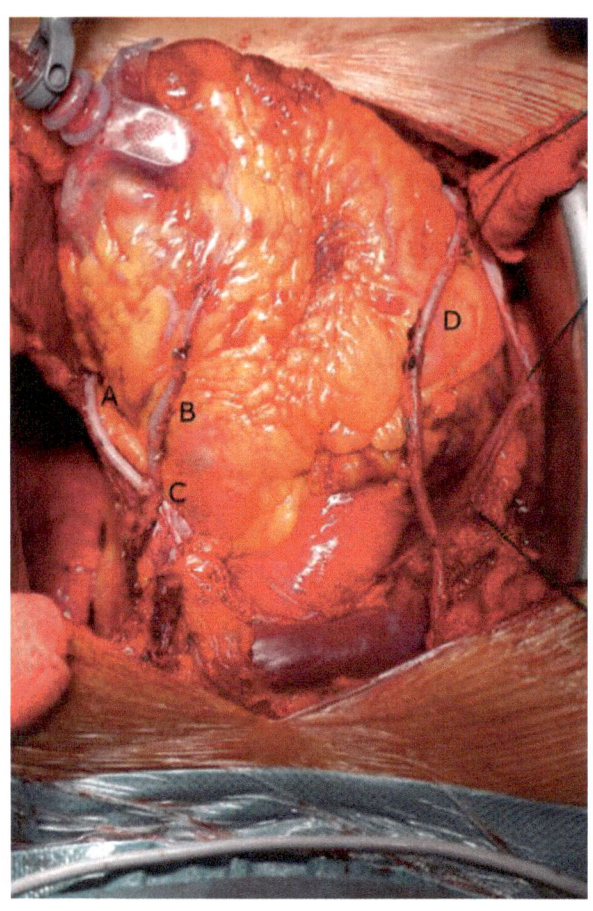

Photo 4.19: LITA to LAD; RA as T-graft to OM; RITA with RA elongation to RPL

*A, RA to OM; B, LITA to LAD; C, T-graft anastomosis; D, RITA with RA elongation to RPL*

### *4.4.3   BITA Composite Variation 1*

(a).  LITA (*in situ*) + RITA (composite)
(b).  LITA (in situ) + sequential RITA (composite)

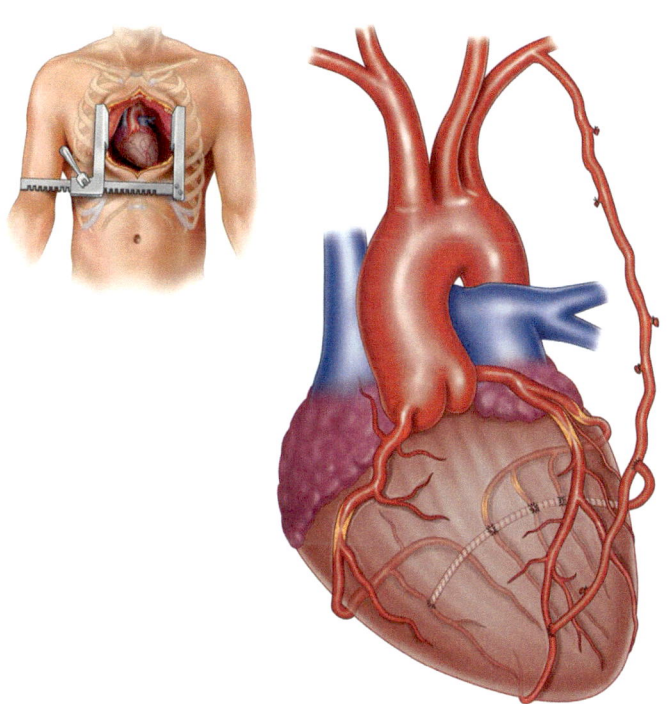

## 4.4.3.1   Prototype Profile

Pragmatic solution for a broad spectrum of patients provid-
ing an anaortic approach and total arterial grafting also in the
presence of complex coronary disease.

| | |
|---|---|
| Age (y) | Young → old |
| Coronary pathology | 2-/3-vessel disease (LAD+CX±RCA), also suitable for small diameter coronaries |
| Residual coronary flow | Low → intermediate (LAD) |
| Complexity of coronary disease | Low → high |
| Urgency | Elective → emergency |
| Operative risk | Low → high |
| Left ventricular function | Normal → low |
| Aortic atherosclerosis | None → complex ("anaortic OPCAB") |
| Co-morbidities | Not exceeding intermediate risk of sternal wound infection |
| Further aspects | Might be reconsidered in very sportive patients (due to single inflow) |
| Bypass material | BITA |

## 4.4.3.2   Prototype Coronary Angiography

Variation 1a:

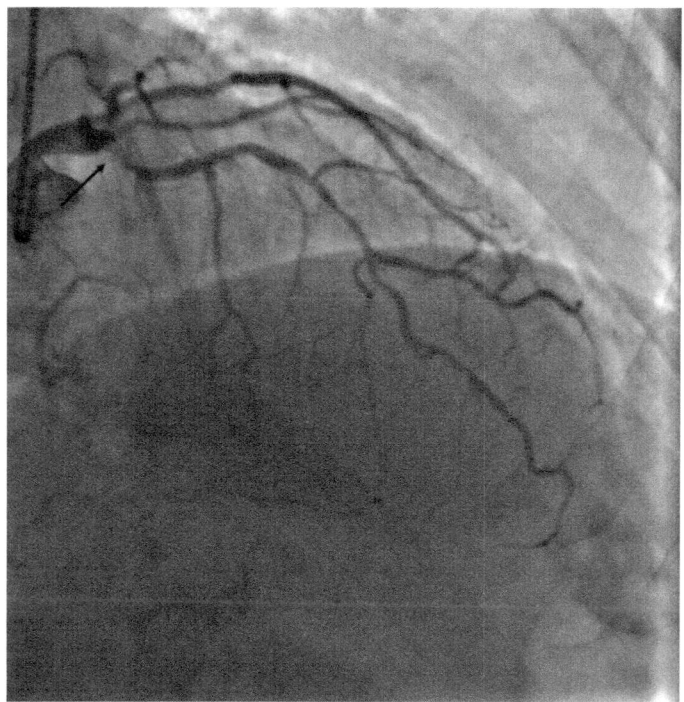

ANGIOGRAM 4.22: Coronary angiogram of the left coronary circulation

→, *LAD stenosis*

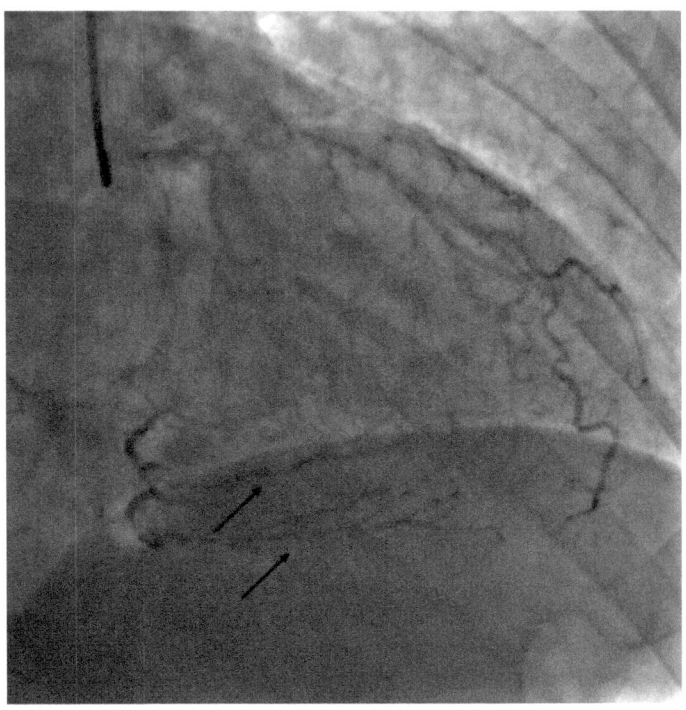

ANGIOGRAM 4.23: Coronary angiogram of the left coronary circulation
→, *collateralized PDA*

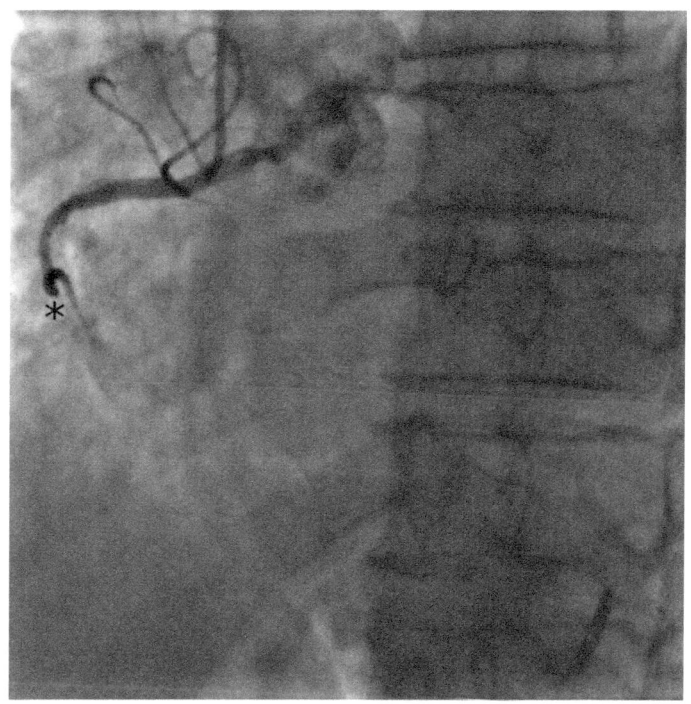

ANGIOGRAM 4.24:  Coronary angiogram of the right coronary circulation
*, RCA CTO

Variation 1b:

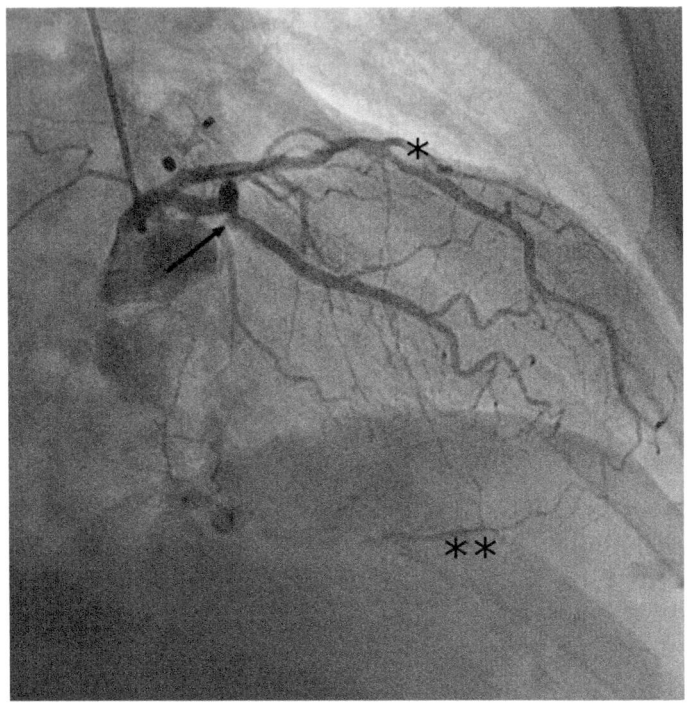

ANGIOGRAM 4.25 Coronary angiogram of the left coronary circulation
→, *CX stenosis; *, LAD stenosis; **, collateralized PDA*

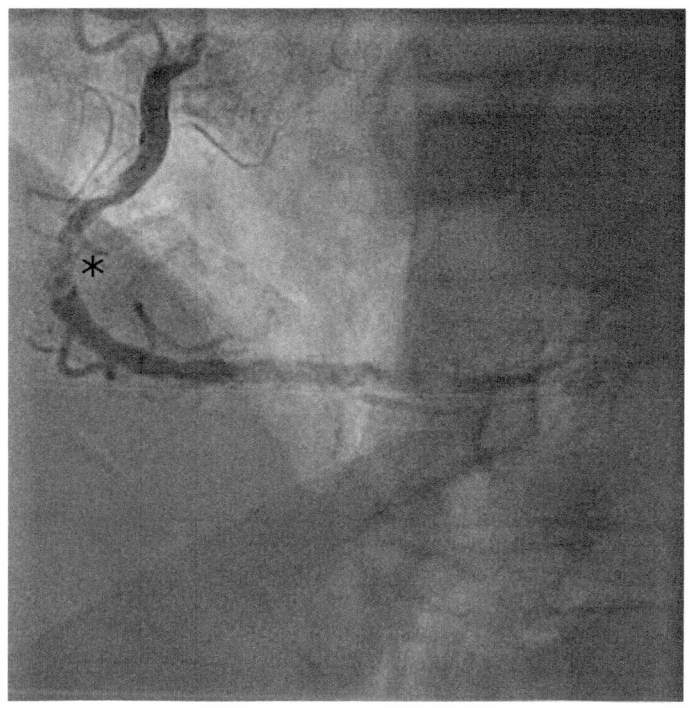

ANGIOGRAM 4.26:  Coronary angiogram of the right coronary circulation
*, RCA stenosis

### 4.4.3.3    Surgical Technique

**Variation 1a: LITA to LAD, RITA as T-graft to PDA**

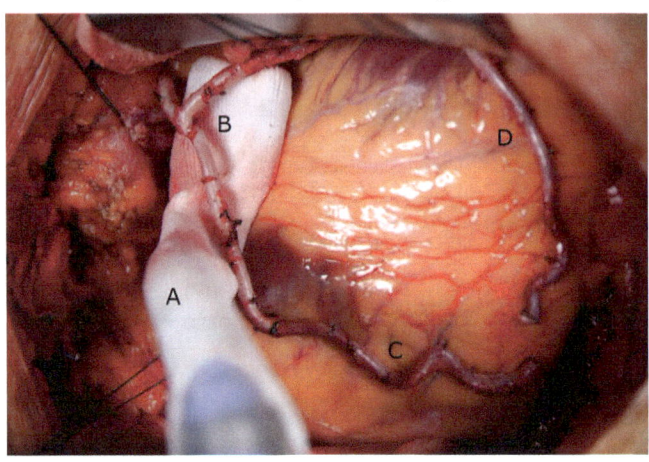

Photo 4.20: T-graft
*A, suction stabilizer; B, T-graft; C, LITA; D, RITA*

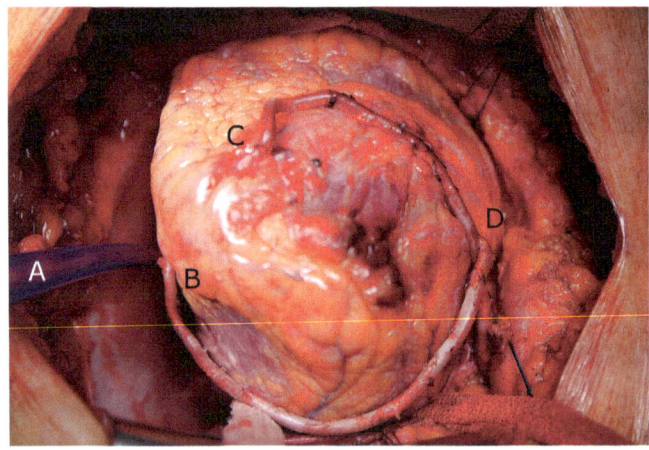

Photo 4.21: LITA to LAD, RITA as T-graft to PDA
*A, deep stitch; B, distal anastomosis RITA to PDA; C, distal anastomosis LITA to LAD; D, T-graft anastomosis*

## Variation 1b: LITA to LAD, RITA as T-graft to OM1 and PDA

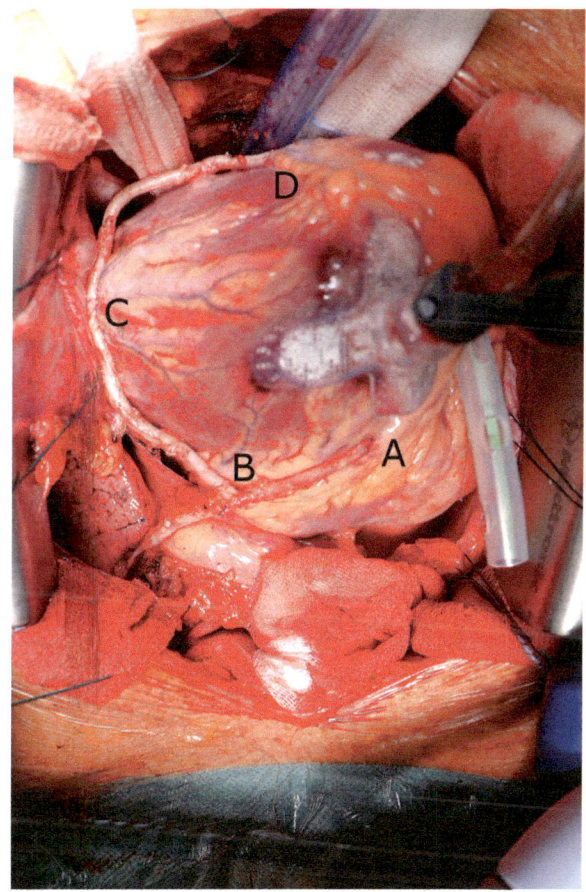

PHOTO 4.22:  LITA to LAD, RITA as T-graft to OM1 and PDA
*A, LITA to LAD; B, T-graft anastomosis; C, RITA to OM1; D, RITA to PDA*

### 4.4.4   BITA Composite Variation 2

LITA (*in situ*) + RITA (composite) + RA/SV (aortic)

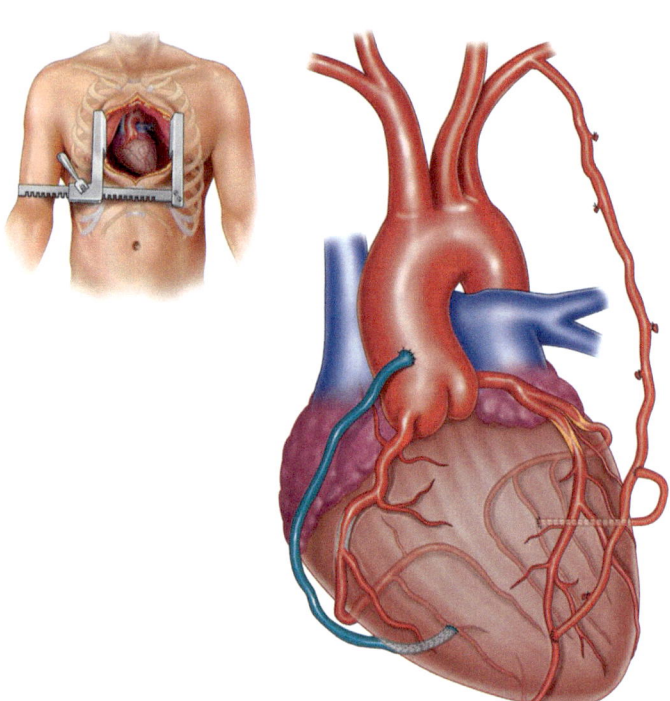

## 4.4.4.1   Prototype Profile

Extended arterial grafting in case of significant competitive RCA flow or in case of insufficient length of the composite RITA.

| | |
|---|---|
| Age (y) | Young → old |
| Coronary pathology | 2-/3-vessel disease (LAD+CX±RCA), also suitable for small diameter coronaries |
| Residual coronary flow | Low (LAD+CX) → intermediate (RCA) |
| Complexity of coronary disease | Low → high |
| Urgency | Elective → emergency |
| Operative risk | Low → high |
| Left ventricular function | Normal → low |
| Aortic atherosclerosis | None → moderate ("clampless OPCAB") |
| Co-morbidities | Not exceeding intermediate risk of sternal wound infection |
| Further aspects | Broad variety of patients |
| Bypass material | BITA and RA/SV |

## 4.4.4.2    Prototype Coronary Angiography

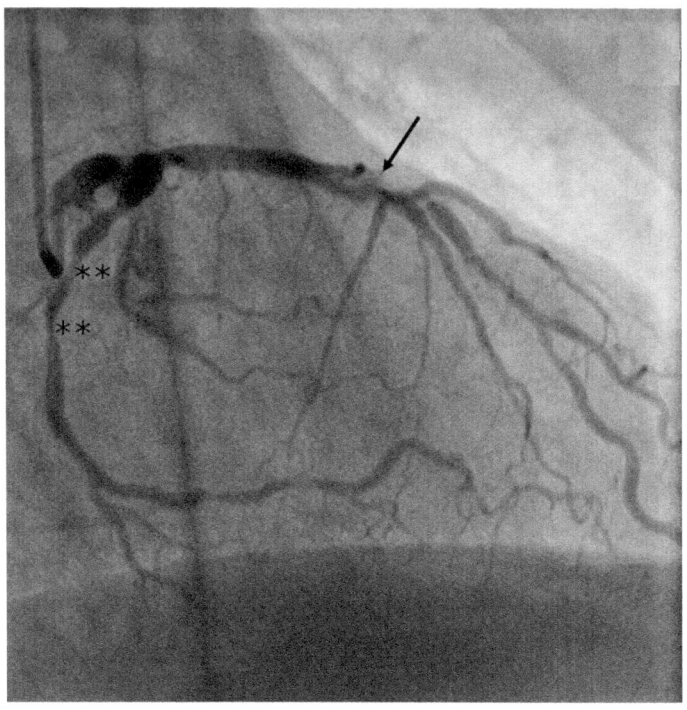

ANGIOGRAM 4.27: Coronary angiogram of the left coronary circulation
→, *LAD stenosis; \*\*, CX stenoses*

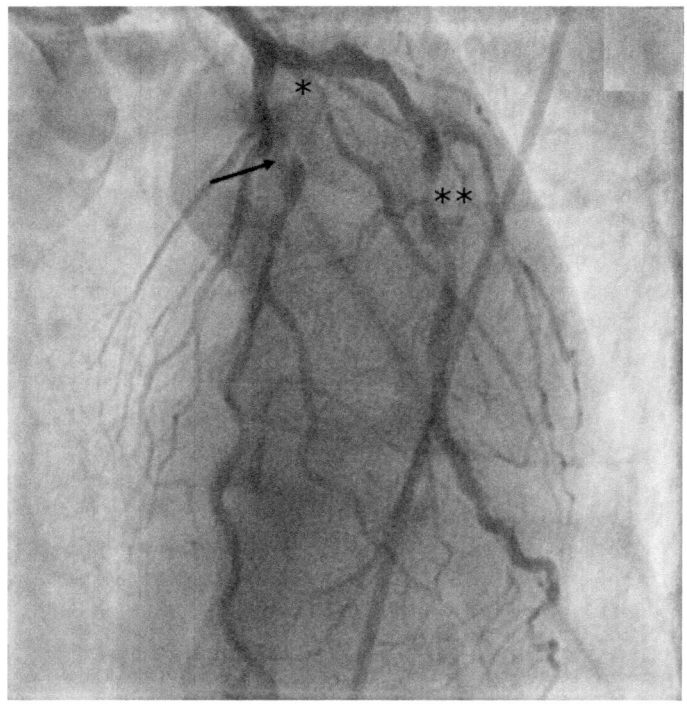

ANGIOGRAM 4.28: Coronary angiogram of the left coronary circulation

→, *LAD stenosis; *, IM stenosis; **, CX stenosis*

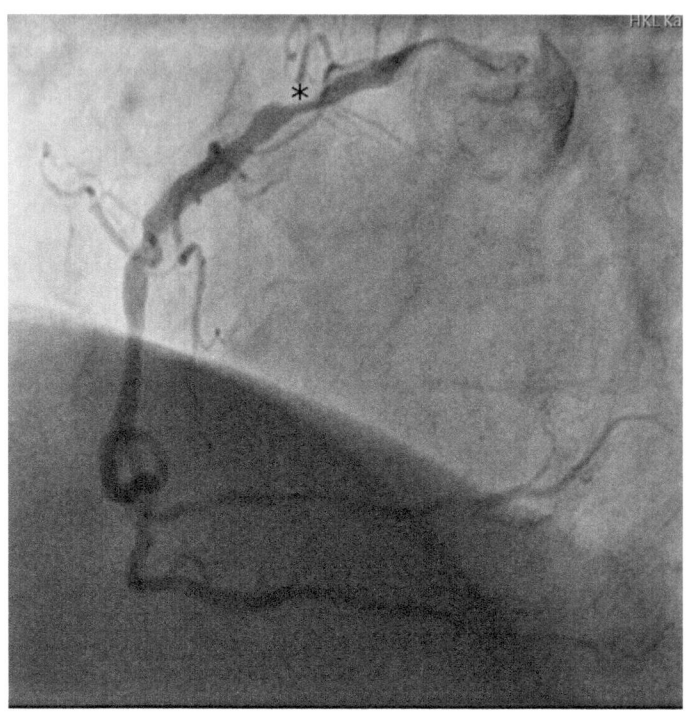

ANGIOGRAM 4.29: Coronary angiogram of the right coronary circulation
*, *RCA stenosis*

## 4.4.4.3   Surgical Technique

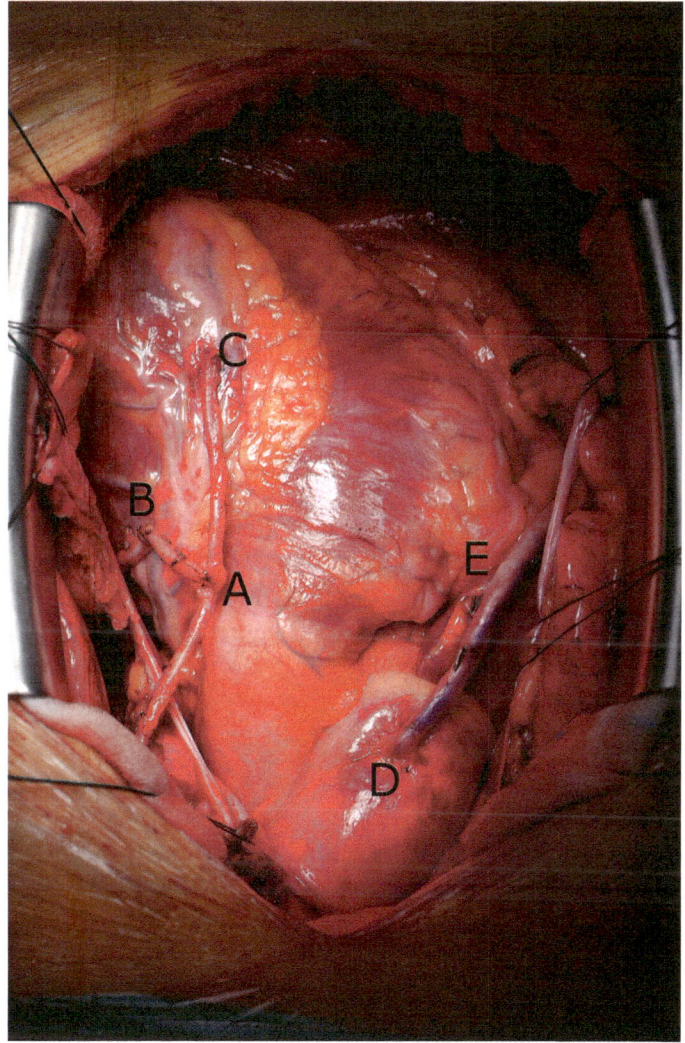

PHOTO 4.23:  LITA to LAD, RITA as T-graft to IM and LPL, SVG to RCA

*A, T-graft anastomosis; B, RITA to IM; C, LITA to LAD; D, aortic anastomosis; E, SVG to RCA*

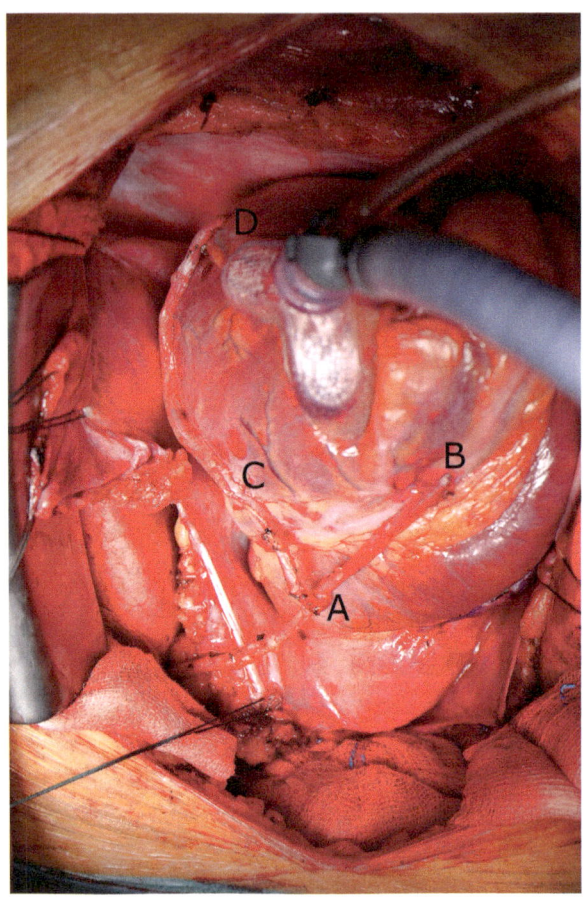

Photo 4.24:  LITA to LAD, RITA as T-graft to IM and LPL, SVG to RCA

*A, T-graft anastomosis; B, LITA to LAD; C, RITA to IM; D, RITA to LPL*

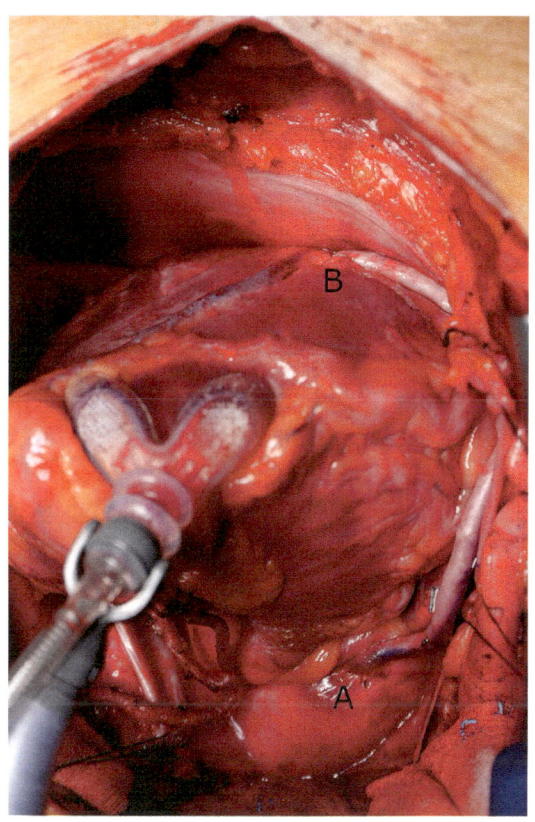

Photo 4.25:  LITA to LAD, RITA as T-graft to IM and LPL, SVG to RCA

*A, aortic anastomosis; B, SVG to RCA*

## 4.5    Single Arterial + Venous Grafting

**Variations:**

1. LITA (*in situ*) + SV (multiple aortic) or LITA (*in situ*) + sequential SV (aortic) (=LITA and SV Variation 1)
2. LITA (*in situ*) + SV (composite) (=LITA and SV Variation 2)

### *4.5.1    LITA and SV Variation 1*

(a).  LITA (in situ) + SV (multiple aortic) or
(b).  LITA (in situ) + sequential SV (aortic)

…according to the surgeon's preference

a

b

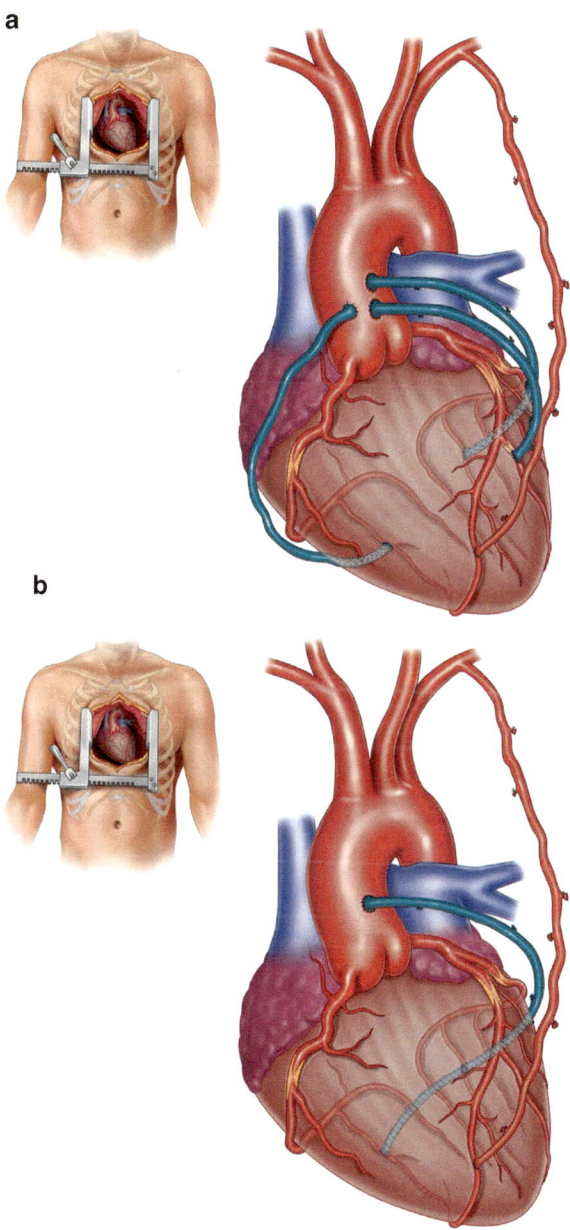

## 4.5.1.1   Prototype Profile

Classical CABG approach for older patients or those with more comorbidities.

| Age (y) | Old |
|---|---|
| Coronary pathology | All 2-/3-vessel disease cases (in small diameter coronaries, sequential arterial grafting might be better) |
| Residual coronary flow | Low → intermediate |
| Complexity of coronary disease | Low → very high |
| Urgency | Elective → emergency |
| Operative risk | Low → high |
| Left ventricular function | Normal → low |
| Aortic atherosclerosis | None → moderate ("clampless OPCAB") |
| Co-morbidities | None → multimorbid patients (alternative: total venous grafting) |
| Further aspects | Broad variety of patients |
| Bypass material | LITA and SV |

## 4.5.1.2    Prototype Coronary Angiography

Variation 1a:

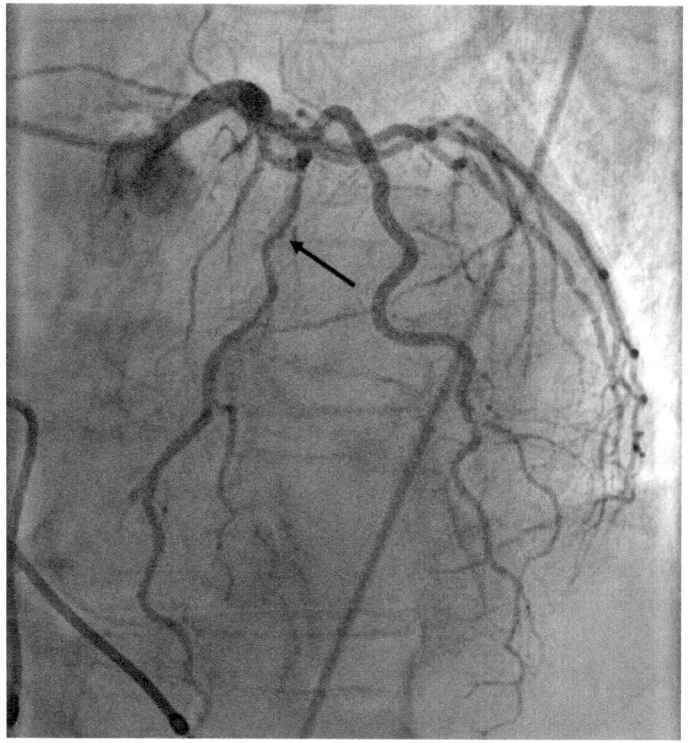

ANGIOGRAM 4.30: Coronary angiogram of the left coronary circulation

→, *LAD stenosis*

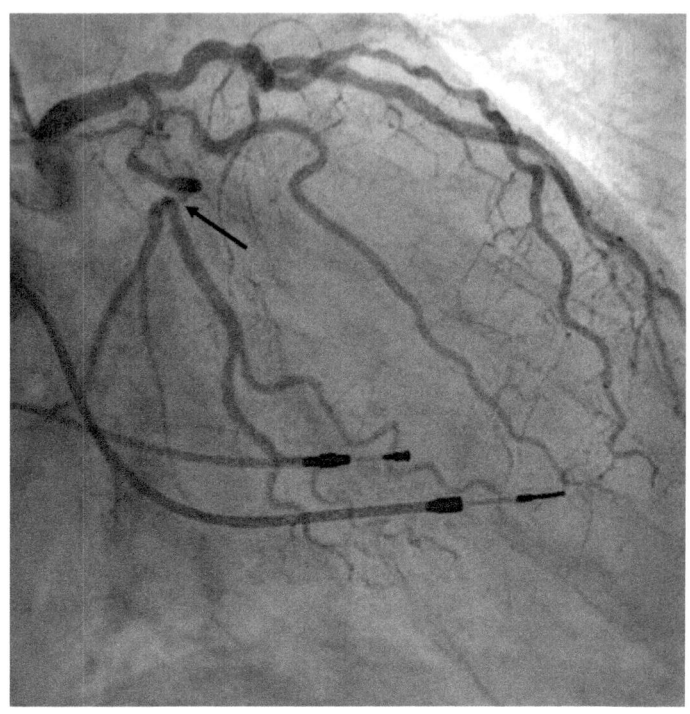

ANGIOGRAM 4.31: Coronary angiogram of the left coronary circulation
→, *CX stenosis*

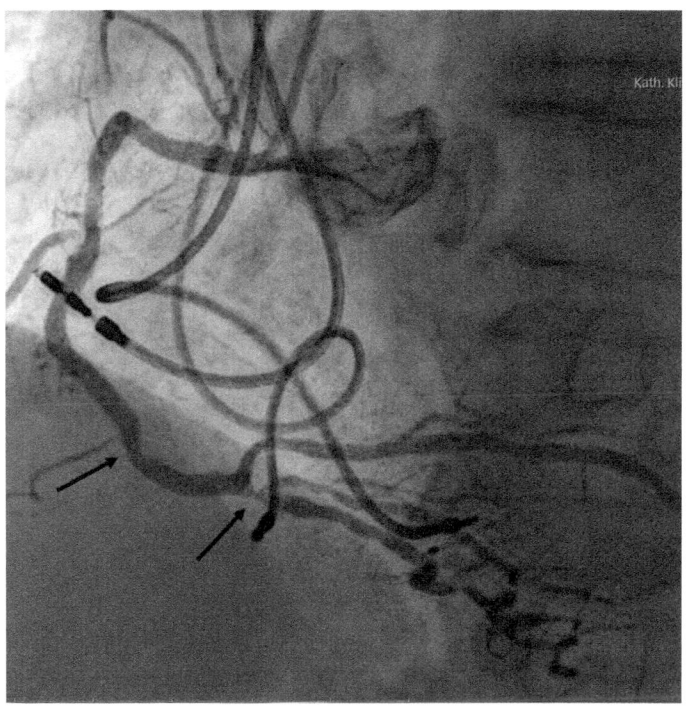

ANGIOGRAM 4.32:  Coronary angiogram of the right coronary circulation

→, *stenoses*

Variation 1b:

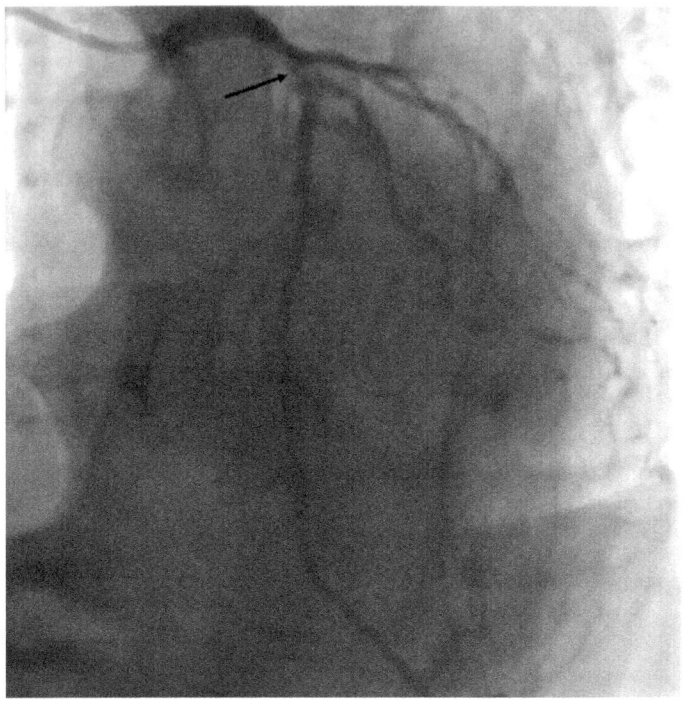

ANGIOGRAM 4.33: Coronary angiogram of the left coronary circulation

→, *LAD stenosis*

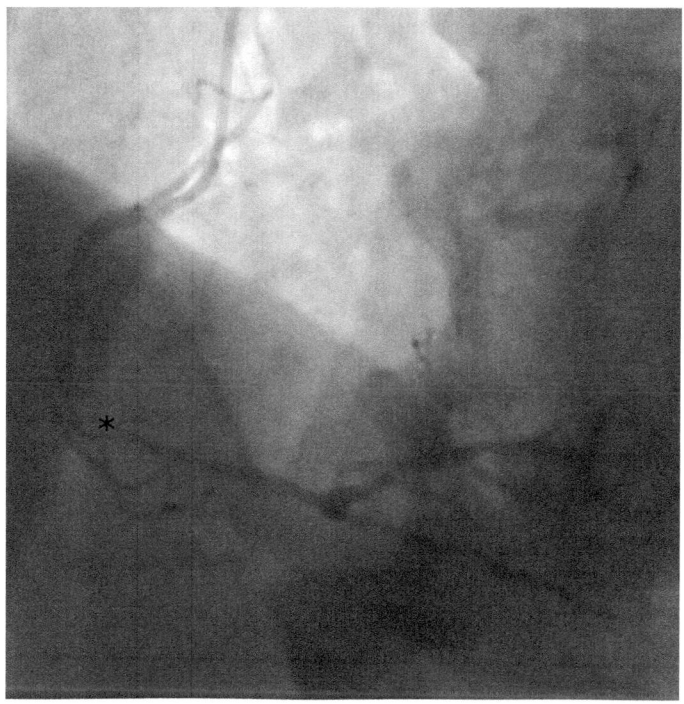

ANGIOGRAM 4.34: Coronary angiogram of the right coronary circulation
*, RCA stenosis

### 4.5.1.3    Surgical Technique

Variation 1a: LITA to LAD, SV to OM2 and sequential SV to PDA and RPL

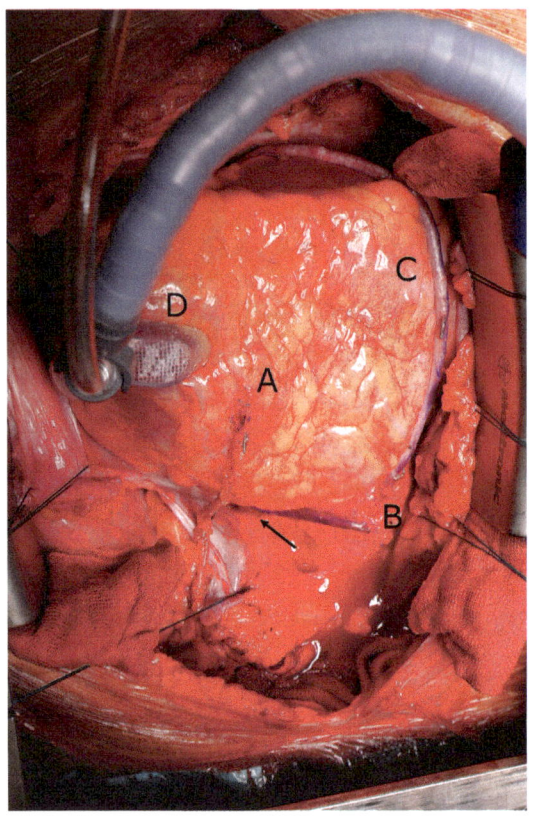

Photo 4.26:  LITA to LAD, SV to OM2 and SV to RPL and PDA
*A, LITA to LAD; B, aortic anastomoses; C, SV to PDA and RPL; D, apically suctioning positioner device; →, SV to OM2*

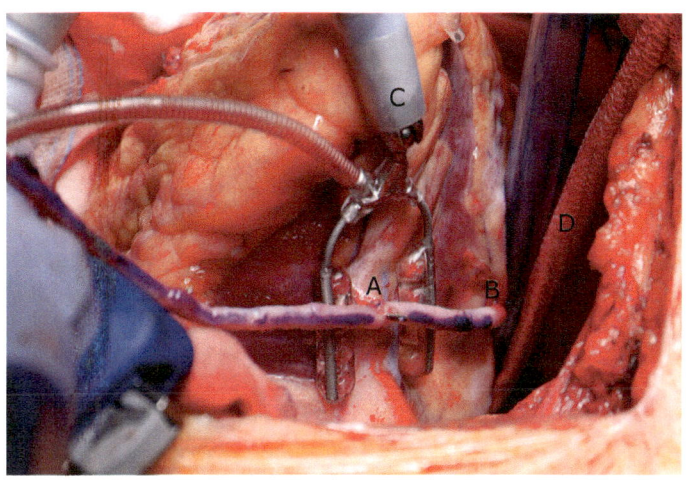

PHOTO 4.27: Detailed picture of the sequential vein graft to RPL and PDA

*A, SV to PDA; B, SV to RPL; C, suction stabilizer; D, deep stitch*

## Variation 1b: LITA to LAD, sequential SV to D, RPL and PDA

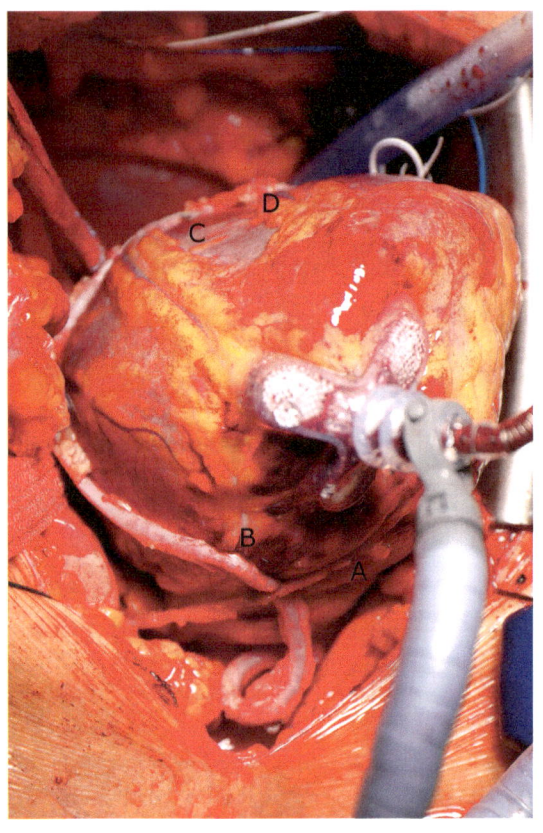

PHOTO 4.28:  LITA to LAD and sequential vein graft to D, RPL and PDA
*A, LITA to LAD; B, SV to D; C, SV to RPL; D, SV to PDA*

## 4.5.2   *LITA and SV Variation 2*

LITA (*in situ*) + SV (composite)

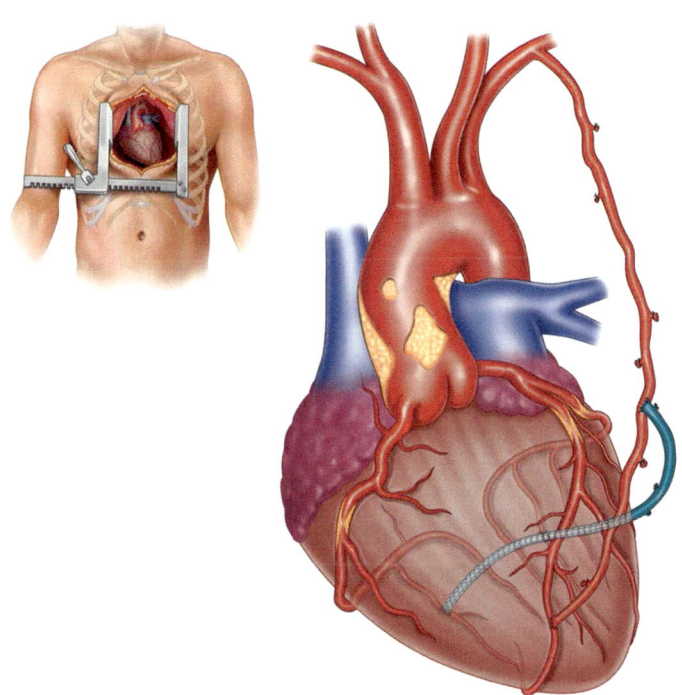

## 4.5.2.1   Prototype Profile

Alternative for patients with high operative risk and severely calcified aorta, but with low risk of competitive flow.

| | |
|---|---|
| Age (y) | Old |
| Coronary pathology | 3-vessel disease (LAD+CX+RCA), high-grade stenoses |
| Residual coronary flow | Low → intermediate (LAD) |
| Complexity of coronary disease | Low → very high |
| Urgency | Elective → emergency |
| Operative risk | Intermediate → high |
| Left ventricular function | Normal → low |
| Aortic atherosclerosis | Complex ("anaortic OPCAB") |
| Co-morbidities | None → multimorbid patients |
| Further aspects | Broad variety of patients |
| Bypass material | LITA and diameter-equivalent SV |

## 4.5.2.2   Prototype Coronary Angiography

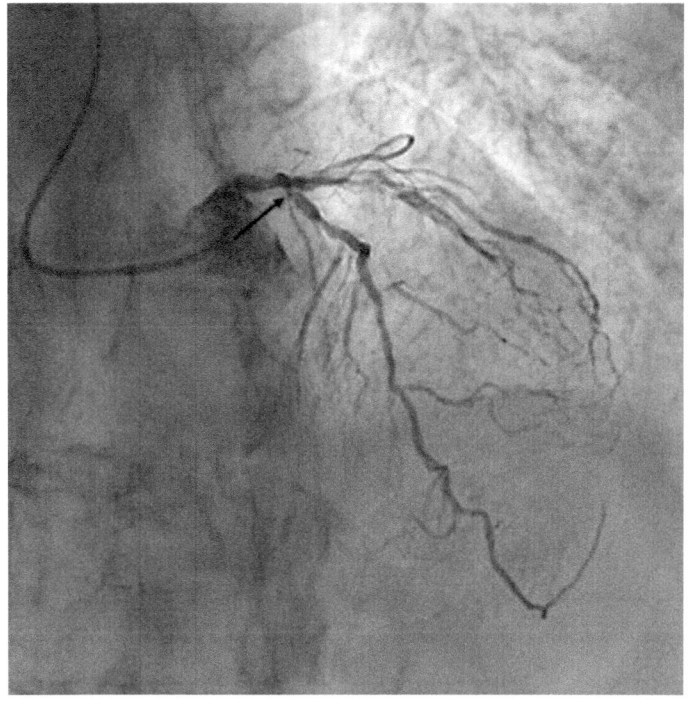

ANGIOGRAM 4.35: Coronary angiogram of the left coronary circulation
→, *LAD stenosis*

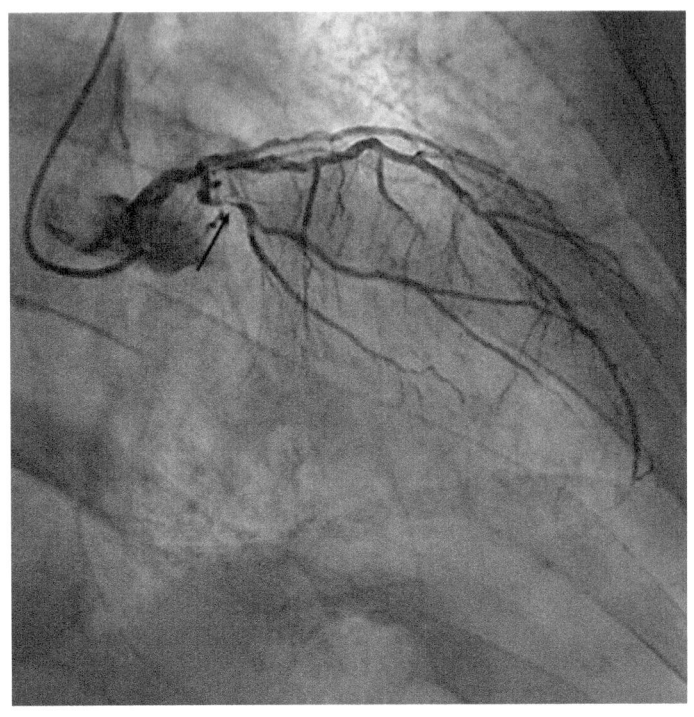

ANGIOGRAM 4.36: Coronary angiogram of the left coronary circulation
→, *CX stenosis*

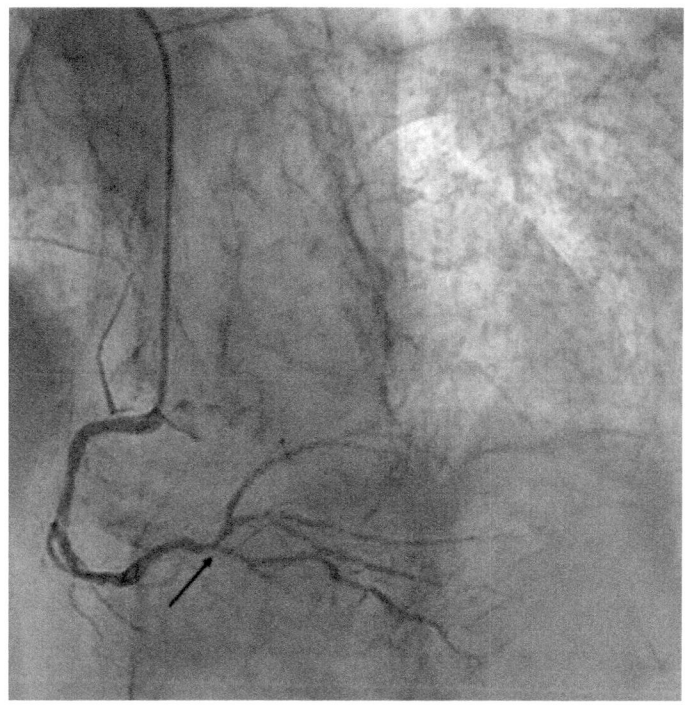

ANGIOGRAM 4.37:  Coronary angiogram of the right coronary circulation
→, *RCA stenosis*

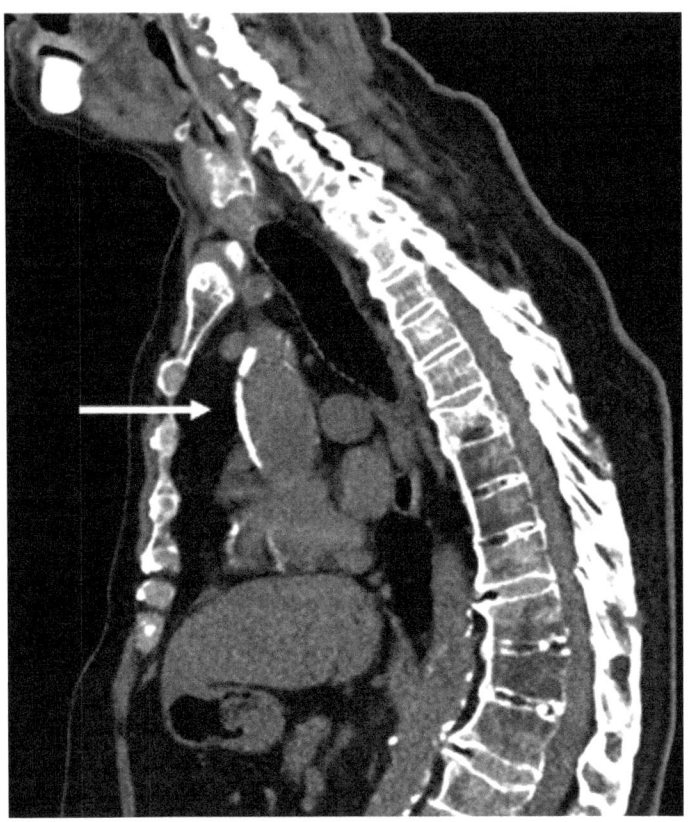

TOMOGRAM 4.1: Computed tomography of the thorax
→, *large anterior plaque in the ascending aorta*

## 4.5.2.3    Surgical Technique

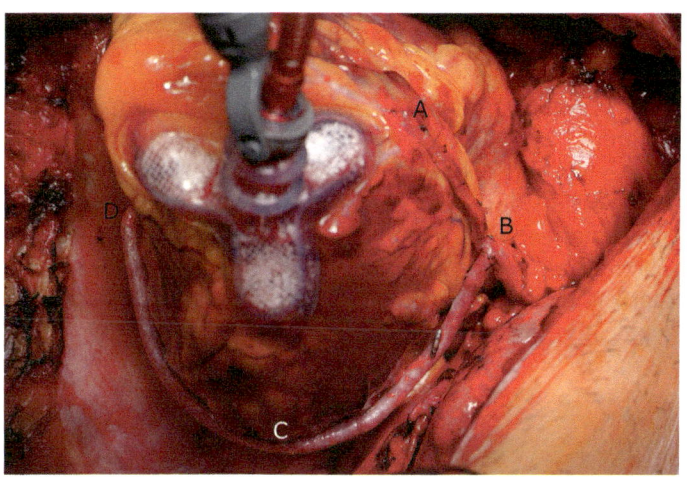

PHOTO 4.29:  LITA to LAD, SV as T-Graft to OM1 and PDA
*A, LITA to LAD; B, T-Graft anastomosis; C, SV to OM1; D, SV to PDA*

# 4.6    On-Pump CABG

## 4.6.1    Prototype Profile

In many patients, CABG can be performed as off-pump or on-pump procedure, whereas non-sternotomy MICS approaches and severe aortic disease require off-pump surgery. On the other side, the availability of heart-lung machines is necessary in emergency cases with ongoing myocardial ischemia, in patients with hemodynamic instability, for revascularization of the CX in the coronary sulcus, and for other technically extremely challenging anastomoses.

## 4.6.2   Surgical Technique

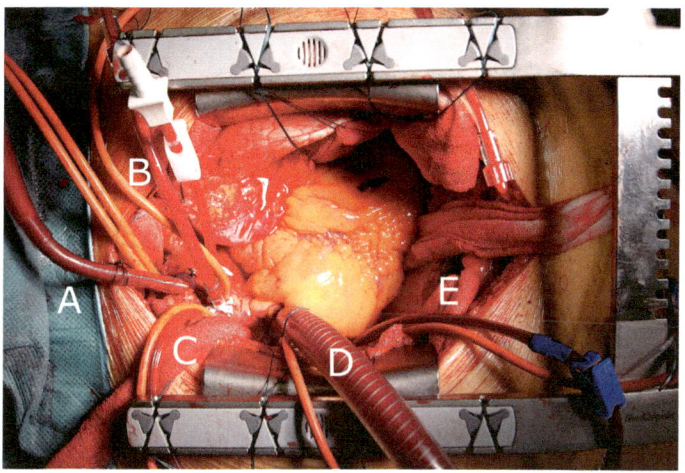

PHOTO 4.30:  On-pump setting
*A, arterial cannula; B, antegrade cardioplegia; C, left ventricular vent catheter; D, venous cannula; E, retrograde cardioplegia*

# Chapter 5
## Perspective MICS-CABG

**M. Marin-Cuartas and P. M. Davierwala**

## 5.1   Introduction

Development and application of minimally invasive cardiac surgery (MICS) has widely expanded over the last two decades [1, 2, 3]. The term "minimally invasive mitral valve surgery" has been traditionally used for mitral valve procedures that are performed through smaller chest wall incisions that avoid a full conventional sternotomy. The current trend and actual purpose of MICS is to avert any form of sternotomy, including partial upper or lower hemi-sternotomy, with the intention to reduce postoperative blood product usage, shorten ventilation times, reduce intensive care and hospital stays, diminish postoperative pain and speed up return to normal physical activities [4]. Although the adoption of MICS techniques has been predominantly applied to valvular heart and single vessel coronary artery bypass graft (CABG) surgery, the last decade has also witnessed a widespread use of minimally invasive techniques for performance of multi-vessel CABG, which is now popularly known as MICS-CABG [5, 6, 7]. The fundamental benefit of MICS-CABG is

M. Marin-Cuartas · P. M. Davierwala (✉)
University Department of Cardiac Surgery, Heart Center Leipzig, Leipzig, Germany

© Springer Nature Switzerland AG 2021                205
A. Albert et al. (eds.), *Operative Techniques in Coronary Artery Bypass Surgery*,
https://doi.org/10.1007/978-3-030-48497-2_5

complete elimination of superficial and deep sternal wound infections and mediastinitis, which is particularly advantageous in patients undergoing BITA grafting. When performed off-pump with composite grafts, MICS-CABG is also associated with a reduction in perioperative stroke rates due to less or no ascending aortic manipulation [8]. In addition, it also provides the patient with other already known benefits of MICS [4]. Nevertheless, MICS-CABG procedures are technically challenging, have a steep learning curve, and require longer operating times. The following chapter offers an overview of the most important aspects related to MICS-CABG. Video-assisted and robotic MICS-CABG are more sophisticated technologies, which are not yet available in most cardiac surgical departments around the world. Therefore, the focus of this chapter will be on MICS-CABG surgery performed under direct visualization through a left mini-thoracotomy.

## 5.2    Brief History

The initial advances in the development of MICS techniques were in the field of mitral valve disease. Introduction of modified CPB circuits, less invasive incisions and long-shafted surgical instruments enabled the performance of safe and efficacious minimally invasive surgery [2, 9, 10, 11, 12]. Thereafter, video-endoscopic MICS through a right mini-thoracotomy as well as voice-controlled and totally robotic cardiac surgery were introduced [13, 14, 15]. The reproducibility of these procedures was well-established in institutions with large thoracoscopic and robotic mitral valve repair programs, which delivered excellent results [2, 16, 17, 18, 19]. These advances motivated and led to the development of the minimally invasive surgical treatment of coronary artery disease. The first steps in that direction were through the pioneering work of Benetti [20], who published his work on the MIDCAB procedure, which involved the grafting of the LAD with the LITA through a left anterior small thoracotomy

(LAST) approach. Thereafter, MIDCAB was adopted by several groups in the mid- 90s [21, 22, 23, 24]. It also gave birth to hybrid coronary revascularization that was first described by Angelini *et al* in 1996 [25] and involves combining a MIDCAB procedure with PCI in selected patients. Expanding the MIDCAB procedure to multivessel CABG through the LAST approach, which involved grafts to the lateral and inferior walls of the heart, took a while before the first report about its feasibility, safety and applicability was published a decade ago [6]. Since then, several groups all over the world have adopted and further developed this MICS-CABG procedure [26, 27, 28, 29, 30, 31].

# 5.3   Patient Selection and Preoperative Screening

All patients with an indication for isolated surgical revascularization may be considered potential candidates for a MICS-CABG approach. Patients requiring isolated left-sided coronary revascularization are, however, ideal candidates for this procedure. It is possible to graft the RCA, but can be technically more challenging. If the surgeon wants to perform the operation without implementation of CPB, it would be advisable to pay heed to certain patient parameters that could help him/her expedite the procedure with greater ease and efficiency, at least in the early phase of his/her experience. Patients with a body-mass index (BMI) <30 kg/m$^2$, a cardiothoracic-ratio (CTR) <50%, left ventricular ejection fraction (LVEF) >45%, left ventricular end-diastolic internal diameter (LVEDID) <55 mm and good coronary targets are favourable candidates for this procedure. In short, the thoracic cavity should have adequate volume to enable mobilization of the heart into various positions required to graft different territories without producing hemodynamic instability. The surgeon does not have the luxury of placing a part of the heart outside of the thoracic cavity as in case of a sternotomy approach. The above-mentioned selection criteria can be relaxed with increasing experience of the operating team. Contrarily, if the operation is performed on CPB with or without the use of aortic clamping, all CABGs can be performed with this approach. However, we believe that avoiding the use of CPB and aortic clamping are of utmost importance in reducing invasiveness of a CABG procedure. Absolute and relative contraindications for off-pump MICS-CABG are summarized in (Table 5.1).

The preoperative assessment includes the usual laboratory tests such as a total blood count, blood sugar levels, serum electrolytes, renal and liver function tests, and a complete coagulation profile, electrocardiography and carotid Doppler sonography that are routinely performed prior to any cardiac surgical procedure. Additionally, a chest X-ray, transthoracic echocardiography, and pulmonary function tests, which are routine in most institutions, should also be performed to assess the selection criteria of the patients for off-pump CABG. We do not perform computed tomographic (CT) scanning of the chest routinely. However, a coronary CT-scan can be useful in locating occluded or anomalous coronary targets not visualized on conventional coronary angiography or in depicting the exact position of deep intramuscular vessels.

# 5.4    Operative Management

## 5.4.1    Intraoperative TEE

The volume status, cardiac performance, and use of vasopressors or inotropes are chiefly assessed and guided by TEE. It is also used to monitor the mitral and tricuspid valves for new-onset or worsening of pre-existing regurgitation and to identify the development of severe right ventricular outflow tract (RVOT) obstruction during subluxation of the heart and new regional wall motion abnormalities, and to help safe insertion and placement of femoral venous and arterial cannulas, in case CPB is required.

TABLE 5.1
Contraindications
for off-pump
MICS-CABG

| *Absolute contraindications* |
| --- |
| Severe obesity |
| COPD (precludes single-lung ventilation) |
| Interstitial lung disease |
| Severe pulmonary hypertension |
| Severe chest deformity |
| Highly stenotic or occluded left subclavian artery |
| Emergent CABG |
| *Relative contraindications* |
| Diffuse CAD |
| Severely calcified coronary targets |
| Deep intramuscular vessels |
| If intraoperative TEE is contraindicated |

*MICS-CABG* minimally invasive multi-vessel coronary artery bypass grafting, *BMI* body mass index, *COPD* chronic obstructive pulmonary disease, *CABG* coronary artery bypass grafting, *CAD* coronary artery disease, *TEE* transesophageal echocardiography

## 5.4.2   Surgical Setup

Our institution policy is to perform total arterial off-pump MICS-CABG without aortic clamping in majority of cases. Our conduits of choice are BITA followed by the radial artery and in exceptional situations venous grafts. Composite grafts are favored to avoid aortic clamping. The following technique focusses on the use of BITA, but can be extrapolated to any graft used in combination with the LITA. The patient is given a 30° right lateral decubitus position, with the right arm positioned laterally at the level of the posterior axillary line in order to have access to the antero-lateral chest wall. The lower body is placed flat to facilitate access for femoral cannulation in the event of conversion from off- to on-pump CABG and/or venous conduit harvest (Fig. 5.1).

A 6 to 8 cm incision is made in the left fourth or fifth inter-costal space, between the midclavicular and anterior axillary lines. A Thoratrak (Medtronic, Minneapolis, Minnesota, USA) rib spreader is inserted and gradually pulled cephalad and toward the left by using a Rultract Skyhook (Rultract, Cleveland, Ohio, USA) or the IMAGate Sternal wire lift (Geister Medizintechnik GmbH, Tuttlingen, Germany) retractor (Fig. 5.2).

The LITA is harvested in a skeletonized fashion from the left subclavian vein to the bifurcation by direct vision with the help of long-shafted instruments and electrocautery blade (Fig. 5.3a and b).

The skeletonized technique not only provides the additional length that may be required in certain cases, but also prevents development of hyperesthesia that may occasionally occur following pedicled LITA harvest. A harmonic scalpel is also a good alternative for surgeons who already have experi-

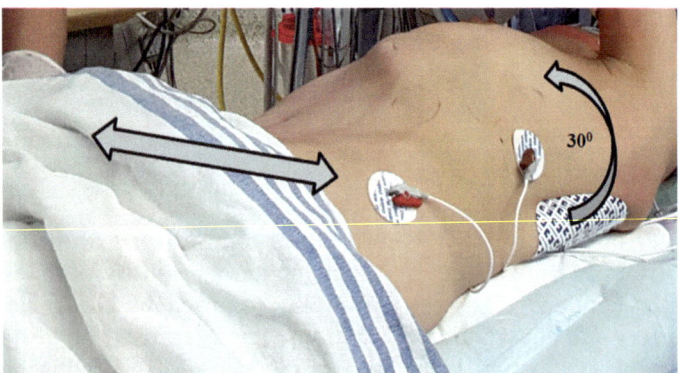

FIGURE 5.1 The patient is given a 30° right lateral decubitus position (curved arrow). The lower body is placed flat (double-headed arrow)

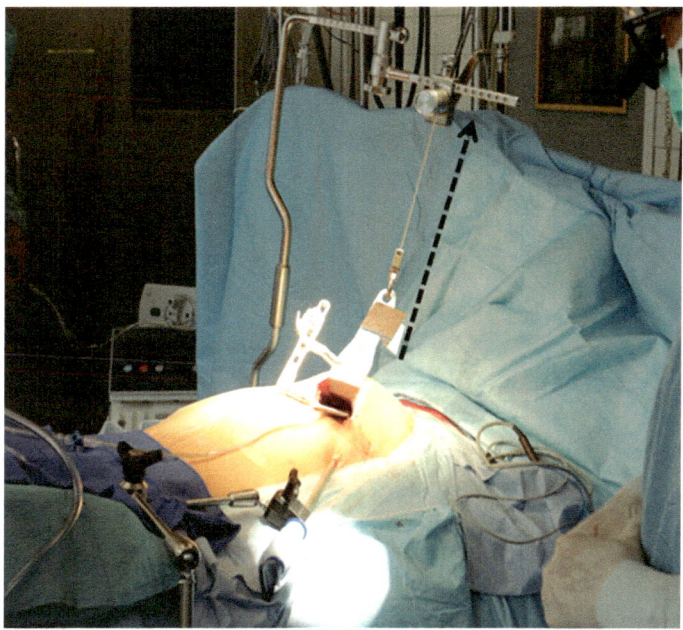

FIGURE 5.2 Thoratrak rib spreader is pulled cephalad and toward the left by the Rultract Skyhook retractor (black hatched arrow)

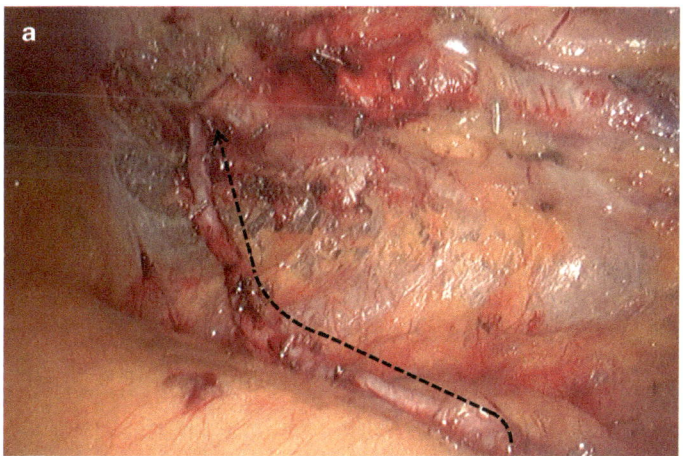

FIGURE 5.3 (**a**) The left internal thoracic artery (ITA) harvest in a skel-etonized fashion (hatched arrow). Distal bifurcation is visualized (arrow-head).

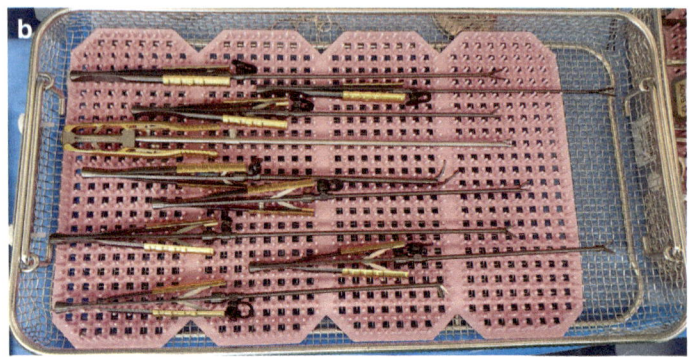

FIGURE 5.3 (**b**) Long-shafted instruments used for harvest of bilateral ITAs

ence with its use. The LITA is transected at its distal end following intravenous administration of 5000 units of Heparin.

Thereafter, dissection of the anterior mediastinum is continued towards the right pleura, which is opened completely. A hook is inserted into the anterior mediastinum under the xyphoid process through a 1 cm subxyphoid incision and connected to an angulated bar, which is fixed to the operating table, with a blade guide and coupling rider (Fehling Surgical Instruments Inc., Karlstein, Germany) and progressively pulled cephalad so that the lower third of the sternum is pulled anteriorly, thereby increasing the space within the thorax to facilitate harvest of the right internal thoracic artery (RITA) (Fig. 5.4).

This maneuver is particularly useful, when the whole length of the RITA is required. When the upper half to three-quarters of the RITA is needed, it suffices to place 3–4 stay sutures into the pericardial fat at the right cardiac border, which are then pulled out through a puncture in the left thoracic wall at the level of the posterior axillary line. Tension on these sutures depresses the tissues anterior to the heart and thus helps increase space in the anterior mediastinum to facilitate RITA harvest (Fig. 5.5).

A laparotomy sponge is inserted into the right pleura to keep the right lung away from the RITA. The RITA can now be visualized clearly and is harvested by direct vision in a skeletonized fashion (Fig. 5.6).

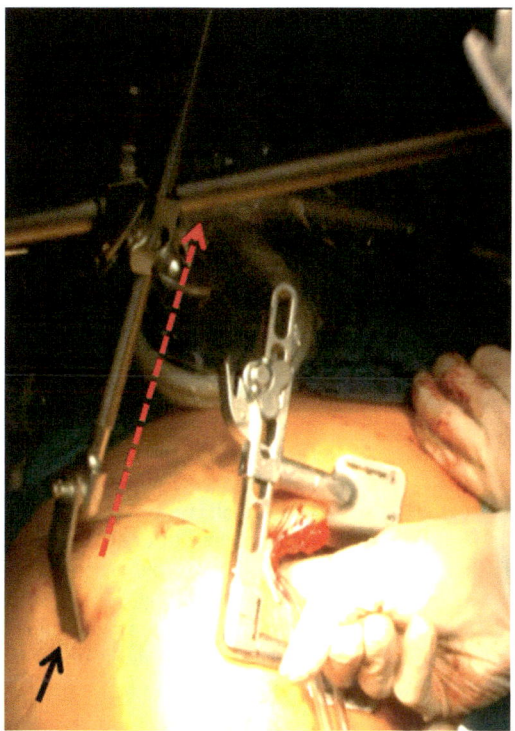

FIGURE 5.4 Sub-xyphoid hook introduced into the anterior mediastinum through a 1 cm subxyphoid incision (black arrow) and pulled cephalad (red hatched arrow) through its connection with an angulated bar

The length of the RITA depends on the number and location of the coronary targets that have to be grafted on the lateral, posterior and lateral walls of the heart. The remaining dose of Heparin is administered intravenous and the RITA is transected proximally and distally for use as a free graft.

The pericardium is then opened in a graded fashion depending on the type of proximal anastomosis to be performed. It is opened anterior to the aorta up to the level of the distal RVOT in patients undergoing a central aortic anastomosis. Several pericardial stay sutures are placed on both sides and are hitched up on to the edges of the thoracotomy incision (Fig. 5.7a). This aids in bringing the aorta as close to

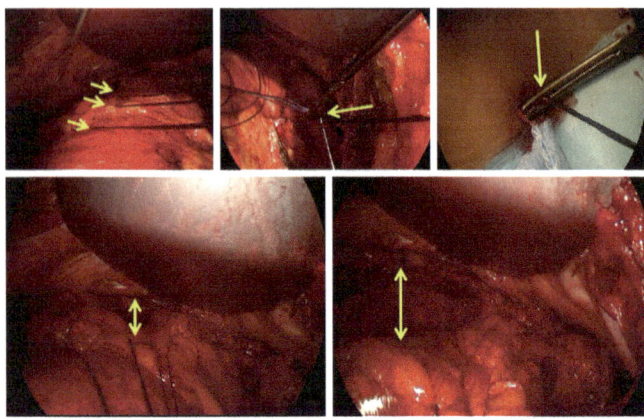

FIGURE 5.5 (**a**) Three stay-sutures in pericardial fat at the right cardiac border (yellow arrows). (**b**) Stay-sutures are grasped by a snare passed through a puncture in the left chest wall (yellow arrow). (**c**) Snare with the stay-sutures are pulled out of the chest through the puncture in the left chest wall (yellow arrow). (**d**) Space in the anterior mediastinum (double-headed yellow arrow) prior to placing the stay sutures under tension. (**e**) Increase in space in the anterior mediastinum (double-headed yellow arrow) after placing the stay sutures under tension

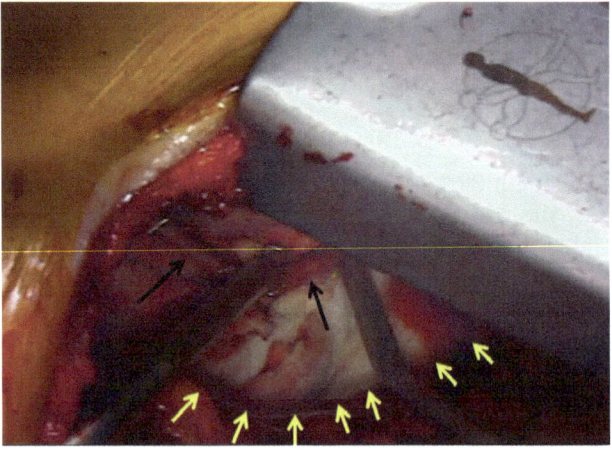

FIGURE 5.6 The right internal thoracic artery (black arrows) harvested in a skeletonized fashion is visualized clearly after placing a white sponge in right pleura (yellow arrows)

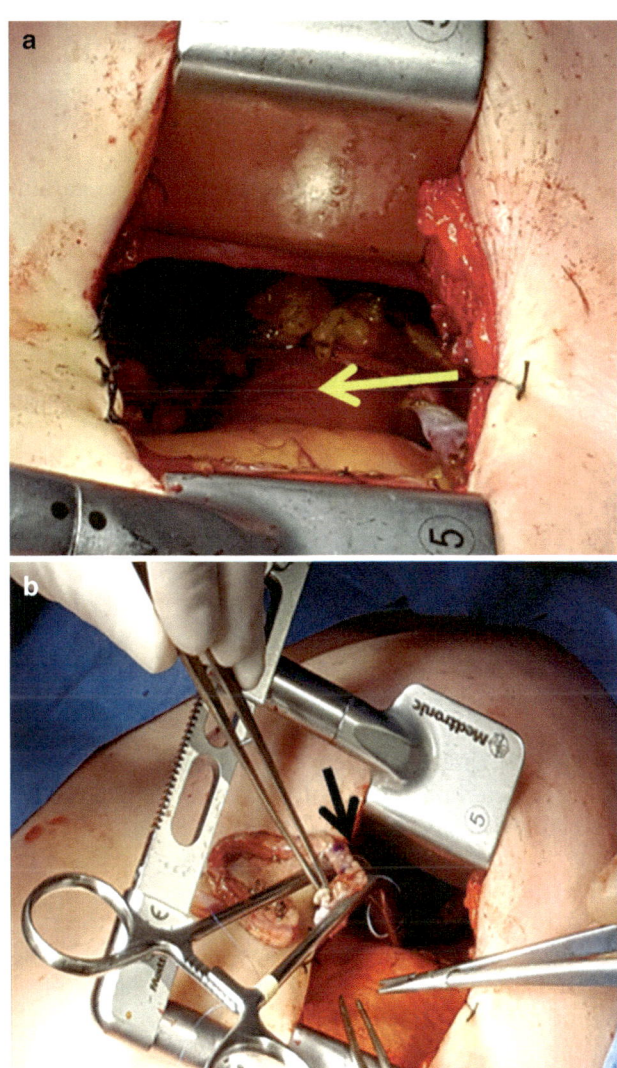

FIGURE 5.7 Proximal anastomosis. (**a**) Several pericardial stay sutures placed on both the edges of the pericardium and hitched up on to the edges of the thoracotomy incision. Yellow arrow shows the ascending aorta. (**b**) The proximal anastomosis performed between the radial artery (black arrow) and ascending aorta with standard instruments in routine fashion

the incision as possible. The proximal anastomosis is then performed with standard instruments in routine fashion, which can be facilitated by a flexible side-biting clamp (Cygnet flexible clamps, Vitalitec, Plymouth, MA, USA) (Fig. 5.7b).

In patients undergoing a Y-anastomosis, the pericardium is first opened from the distal ascending aorta superiorly to about 3–4 cm inferior to the main pulmonary artery. The Y-anastomosis between the LITA and other arterial or venous conduits is constructed at the level of the pulmonary valve. A 5 mm incision is made one or two intercostal spaces inferior to the thoracotomy. An Octopus NS (Medtronic, Minneapolis, Minnesota, USA) epicardial tissue stabilizer is inserted into the left thoracic cavity. The foot pods are covered with a finger glove and are positioned and fixed at the level of the pulmonary valve lateral to the main pulmonary artery. This provides a stable platform to construct the Y-anastomosis (Fig. 5.8a). The proposed spot for the Y-anastomosis on the LITA is fixed to the finger glove with a couple of 6-0 polypropylene sutures, following which, an end-to-side anastomosis is performed with 8-0 polypropylene (Fig. 5.8b).

The Y-anastomosis is then fixed to the lateral wall of the pulmonary trunk at the level of the pulmonary valve and is used as the reference point for measuring the length of the LITA to the LAD or diagonal and the length of the other conduit to the site of the first lateral wall anastomosis (Fig. 5.9).

Thereafter, the pericardium is further opened towards the apex till the LAD is adequately exposed. The anastomotic site is stabilized with the Octopus NS and an end-to-side anastomosis is performed between the LITA and the LAD or a diagonal with 7-0 or 8-0 polypropylene (Fig. 5.10).

Visualization is facilitated by use of an intracoronary shunt and a blower-mister. Thereafter, the high lateral wall vessels such as the intermediate and proximal obtuse marginal arteries are similarly grafted.

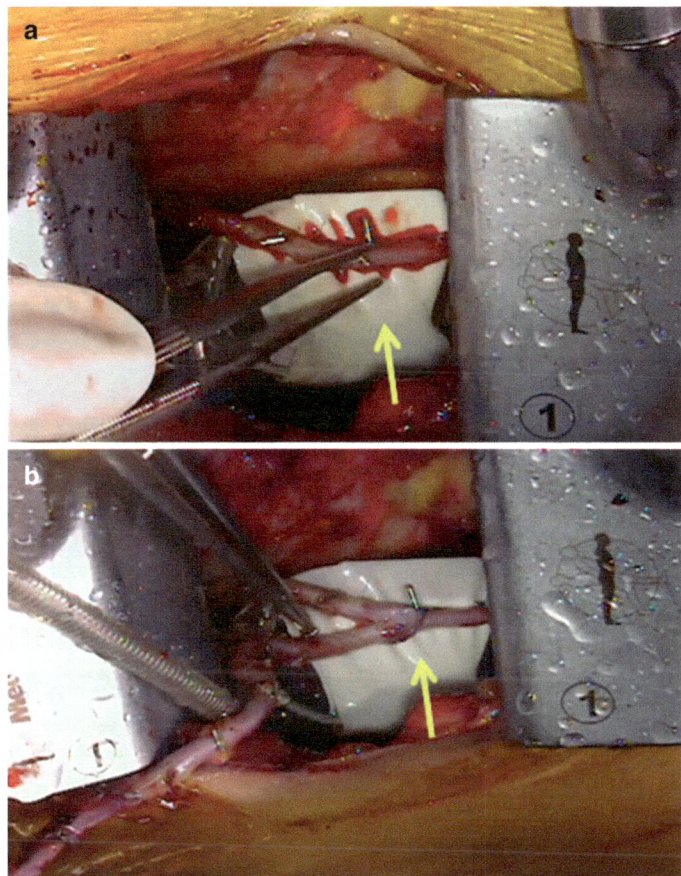

FIGURE 5.8 (**a**) Left internal thoracic artery (yellow arrow) fixed to the finger glove covering pods of the Octopus Nuvo. (**b**) Completed Y-anastomosis between the left and right internal thoracic arteries (yellow arrow)

The pericardiotomy is then extended around the apex of the heart up to the left phrenic nerve. A heart positioner, which enables mobilization of the heart for grafting distal vessels on the posterolateral wall such as the

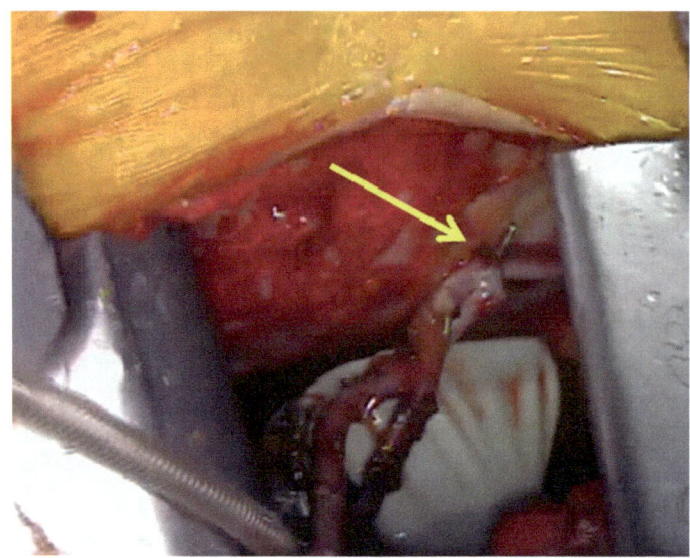

FIGURE 5.9 The Y-anastomosis is fixed to the lateral wall of the pulmonary artery at the level of the pulmonary valve (yellow arrow)

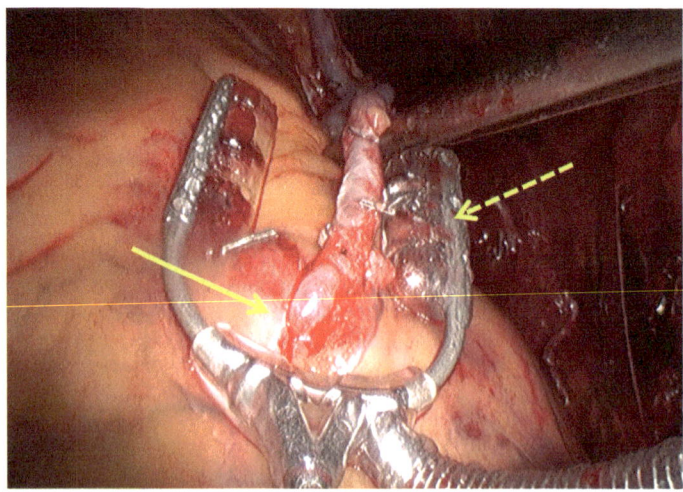

FIGURE 5.10 Left internal thoracic artery—Left anterior descending artery anastomosis (yellow arrow). Foot pods of the Octopus Nuvo stabilizer shown with a yellow hatched arrow

distal obtuse marginal or circumflex or posterolateral ventricular arteries and the posterior descending artery, is utilized. An armless Starfish (Medtronic, Minneapolis, Minnesota, USA) apical positioner with a thick ligature tied to its neck is placed on the appropriate surface of the heart (Fig. 5.11).

The ligature helps in positioning the heart in a way that helps deliver the target vessel as close to the thoracotomy as possible, without causing hemodynamic instability. The apex is pulled towards and under the medial end of the thoracotomy incision for the distal obtuse marginal and circumflex arteries and towards the left shoulder for the posterior descending and distal right coronary arteries. The anastomotic sites on the target vessels have to be further stabilized with the Octopus Nuvo stabilizer (Fig. 5.12).

The anastomoses between the second conduit and the coronary vessels are then performed in a routine manner.

Transit Time Flow Measurement (Medistim) is used to assess the flows in al grafts. Approximately 75% of the calculated dose of protamine is then administered. Thereafter, the heart is returned to its normal position and the pericardium is partially closed over the lower third of the heart, taking precautions to prevent graft kinking or compression. The redundant pericardial fat is further used to cover the anterolateral surface of the heart, in order to prevent displacement of the grafts following inflation of the left lung. Left and right pleural drains are inserted into the thorax through insertion sites of the Octopus Nuvo and subxyphoid hook, respectively. Visualization of the left lung during re-inflation is essential to prevent inadvertent displacement/avulsion of the LITA. The ribs are approximated with a 2-0 polydioxanone suture following intramuscular administration of bupivacaine in 1or 2 intercostal spaces superior and inferior to the thoracotomy. The pectoralis major muscle is approximated with No. 2 polyglactin 910. The subcutaneous tissues and skin are closed in layers.

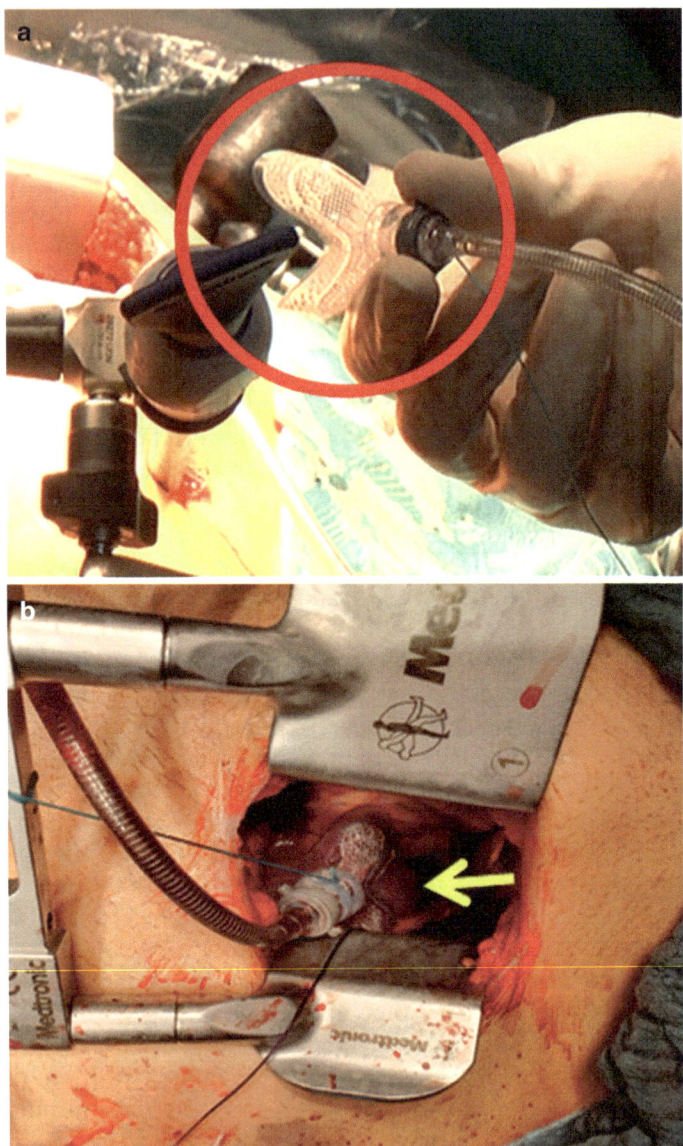

Figure 5.11 (**a**) Armless starfish with a ligature tied to its neck (red circle). (**b**) Armless starfish placed on the lateral wall (not the apex) of the heart for exposure of the high obtuse marginal vessel (yellow arrow)

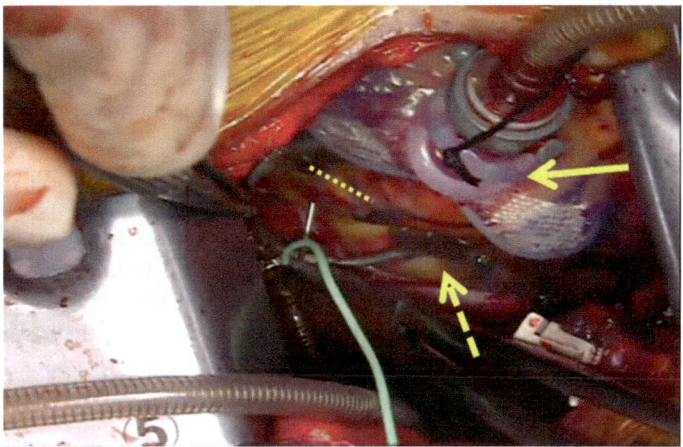

FIGURE 5.12 Positioning for the left circumflex artery anastomosis. Starfish pulls the heart anteriorly (yellow arrow) and the Octopus Nuvo (yellow hatched arrow) stabilizes the target vessel (yellow hatched line)

## 5.5   Tricks and Caveats

Patients undergoing MICS-CABG require single-lung ventilation for prolonged periods of time, extending up to 3–4 h. Therefore, intraoperative lung protective ventilation is paramount in order to prevent lung injury and postoperative respiratory failure. The tidal volume is maintained at 6 ml/kg of the predicted body weight with a positive end expiratory pressure of 5–8 cm $H_2O$. The plateau-pressure is, however, not allowed to exceed 25 cm $H_2O$, and respiratory rate is adjusted to maintain a $PaCO_2 < 5.8$ kPa. Peak inspiratory and driving pressures are also considered for optimizing ventilation and recruitment manoeuvres. The target $SpO_2$ during the entire procedure should be >92% and can be achieved by adjusting the $FiO_2$ between 60–100%. Femoral cannulation can be used if CPB has to be established. During the initial period of ones learning experience, it is advisable to prepare the left femoral vein and artery for cannulation through a small 2 cm groin incision. Once the learning curve has been circumvented, this safety net may not be necessary. Single lung ventilation is not tolerated well by patients suffering from interstitial lung disease or severe pulmonary hypertension. Such patients are not the ideal candidates for a MICS-CABG operation. In contrast, mild to moderate pulmonary emphysema, actually facilitates the operation due to the availability of larger intrathoracic volume for cardiac mobilization. CTR is of utmost importance for off-pump MICS-CABG, because it gives the surgeon a good idea about the relation between the size of the heart and the available intrathoracic space. A CTR <50% facilitates intraoperative heart positioning without hemodynamic instability. Similarly, patients with LVEDID <50 mm and good left ventricular function are generally more suitable for this operation. The potential for torqueing a graft is much higher in patients undergoing MICS-CABG, especially when a large distance exists between two sequential anastomoses. It commonly occurs in patients in whom the heart has to be forced back into its original position at the end of the operation. In such cases, it is recommended to check the position of the graft more than once to rule out a twist, kink or a torque. Since off-pump MICS-CABG is technically challenging, it is essential to monitor graft function before discharge at least in the initial phase of one's experience, so that corrective measures can be implemented when necessary.

## 5.6    Benefits and Drawbacks

MICS-CABG offers all the usual benefits of other MICS procedures such as a decline in blood product usage, shortening of ventilation times and intensive care and hospital stays [4]. However, an important aspect that differentiates MICS-CABG from other MICS procedures is that it can be performed by avoiding CPB and aortic clamping, which we believe is an important aspect of the "minimally invasive" principle for CABG surgery. This is possible by means of off-pump surgery and total arterial revascularization (i.e. BITAs or LITA and RA) with composite grafts, which avoids ascending aortic manipulation, thereby preventing or at least reducing perioperative stroke rates [8, 32]. Reported stroke rates after standard CABG range from 0.6 to 4% [27, 33, 34, 35]. Even in other MICS-CABG series, in which aortic manipulation was not avoided, stroke rates ranged between 0.4 and 0.6% [6, 36]. Contrarily, our MICS-CABG cohort of 88 patients undergoing BITA grafting had no stroke or neurological complications [28], which correlates well with the results reported by Lemma et al., who also reported no neurological complications after MICS-CABG with a composite Y/T-graft constructed with the LITA and radial artery or saphenous vein [37]. Another factor that may play a role in the lower incidence of peri-procedural stroke rates is the relatively low incidence of postoperative atrial fibrillation (AF) associated with MICS procedures, such as minimally invasive mitral valve surgery [4, 10, 38]. AF is known to be an independent predictor for the development of perioperative stroke (HR:4.1;95%CI:1.9–8.8; $P$ = 0.0003) [39]. Our MICS-CABG cohort had an AF rate of 14.8%, which is lower than patients undergoing PCI or standard CABG [39]. Furthermore, utilization dual antiplatelet therapy with aspirin and clopidogrel for 6 months following MICS-CABG in all our patients also could have helped in countering the hypercoagulability that is often observed after off-pump CABG [40].

A large body of evidence supports the use of multiple arterial grafting for improving patient survival following CABG [41]. The use of BITAs is associated with improved survival and freedom from coronary reinterventions, the benefit being even higher in the second decade after surgery [42, 43]. Nevertheless, increased prevalence of sternal wound infections and reconstructions following CABG continues to be the Achilles' heel of BITA use [44]. MICS-CABG spares the sternotomy, thus allowing the use of BITAs without the sternal wound problems. Additionally, superficial and deep chest wound infections affecting the thoracotomy site are also rare [6, 32, 39, 40].

One of the most important advantages of MICS-CABG is the early recovery of patients and return to normal physical activity that is much sooner than for conventional CABG through a sternotomy. In both, the SYNTAX and FREEDOM trials [45, 46], CABG was shown to have statistically significant lower angina score on the Seattle Angina Questionnaire (SAQ) scale than PCI at and beyond 6 months of follow up, with positive impacts on quality of life. However, at 1 month follow-up in the SYNTAX and 1- and 6-month follow-up in the FREEDOM trial, the CABG group had significantly lower SF-36 Physical Component Summary (PCS) score and EQ-5D utilities as well as significantly lower score in the three components of the SAQ, respectively, compared to the PCI group, thereby reflecting the invasiveness of sternotomy CABG and demonstrating that sternotomy CABG patients suffer significantly in the first 6 months [45, 47]. Several observational studies comparing MICS-CABG to sternotomy CABG have consistently shown earlier recovery for MICS-CABG surgery with respect to significantly shorter median length of hospital stay as well as shorter median time to return to full physical activity [48, 49]. The Minimally Invasive coronary surgery compared to STernotomy coronary artery bypass grafting Randomized Control Trial, which is an ongoing multicenter study aimed at assessing quality of life and recovery in patients undergoing sternotomy CABG or MICS CABG early after surgery, will probably provide the evidence in favor or against non-sternotomy approaches [50].

The detractors of MICS-CABG argue that the potential for incomplete revascularization (IR) is higher with the minimally invasive technique in comparison to conventional CABG. Nevertheless, this assumption is based only on the technical complexity of MICS-CABG procedures and is not supported by scientific evidence. In our series of 88 patients, the rate of IR was only 4.5% and was primarily due to non-graftable chronically occluded vessels, which typically have severely fibrotic thick walls and very small lumen [28]. Similarly, McGinn et al. reported a 95% rate of completeness of revascularization in the first 450 patients undergoing minimally invasive multi-vessel CABG[6]. When compared to major randomized controlled trials, IR rates in our series were much lower than those observed in the off- and on-pump patient cohorts of the ROOBY (17.8% and 11.1%), CORONARY (11.8% and 10.0%) and the SYNTAX trials (36.8%) [33, 34, 35]. This could be attributed to the importance given to coronary anatomy as a major criterion in the selection process of patients for this operation. The suitability of coronary anatomy for achieving complete revascularization through MICS-CABG should be at the discretion of the operating surgeon and should be determined based on the experience of the operating team. Additionally, MICS-CABG further provides a good platform for achieving complete revascularization through preplanned hybrid procedures in select patients who have RCA lesions that are amenable to PCI with excellent expected long-term patency.

Another possible argument against MICS-CABG surgery could be that the quality of anastomoses may not be comparable to that performed during conventional CABG. We, therefore, performed a pre-discharge coronary angiography in all patients during the initial phase of our experience to assess the quality of the grafts and the anastomoses. We found a 97% patency rate for both the LITA and the RITA [28]. Ruel et al. also reported an overall graft patency of 92% (LITA graft patency: 100% and saphenous vein graft patency: 85%) on CT angiography performed 6 months following MICS-CABG [51]. Both above-mentioned studies included the learning curves of the surgeons as well. One of the factors that could have attributed to our satisfactory postoperative graft patency could be the use of dual antiplatelet therapy that can offset the hypercoagulability associated with off-pump CABG [40, 52].

Another potential drawback that one could foresee following off-pump MICS-CAG surgery, especially when performed with BITAs, is an increase in respiratory insufficiency. Contrary to expectations, single-lung ventilation for prolonged periods of time (3–4 h in some cases) did not lead to increased respiratory failure rates in our patients (5.7%). This finding is consistent with that reported in the CORONARY trial (5.9% for off-pump group) [33], as well as a 5.8% respiratory failure rate observed by McGinn et al. in their series of 450 patients undergoing MICS-CABG [6]. As described above, lung-protective ventilation is important to prevent this complication.

Postoperative pain is another probable disadvantage in patients undergoing MICS, predominantly due to rib-spreading. Pain has been mostly shown to be equivalent to a full sternotomy approach for the first two postoperative days, with a significant reduction thereafter [9]. Studies have also demonstrated that patients who underwent a MICS as a reoperation felt that their recovery was more rapid and less painful than after their original sternotomy procedure [16, 53]. However, rib-spreading during MICS-CABG can be associated in few cases with greater postoperative pain than a midline sternotomy due to the greater amount of rib-spreading that is necessary in comparison to minimally invasive valve procedures. However, in our series, only three patients required patient controlled analgesia, which is offered to patients who have severe unrelenting pain that is not responsive to opioid analgesics and corresponds to level 4–5 out of 10 on the pain scale. Gradual progressive spreading of the ribs during ITA harvest in order to prevent rib fractures as well as splitting of the pectoralis major muscle well beyond the ends of the skin incision may contribute to a reduction in pain levels following MICS-CABG. Additionally, we routinely inject the intercostal spaces adjacent to the incision with bupivacaine.

## 5.7    Learning Curve

MICS-CABG is associated with a steep learning curve not only for the surgeon but also for the entire surgical team. The anaesthesiologist has to learn special ventilator maneuvers that not only help maintain adequate oxygenation and $CO_2$ elimination, but also help the surgeon in achieving and maintaining a heart position which provides adequate exposure of grafting target vessels without leading to hemodynamic instability. Furthermore, the surgeon has to adapt to a limited surgical field and restricted movements while performing distal anastomoses. Finally, the assistant surgeon and surgical nurse have to get accustomed to unconventional instruments and to assist with limited vision. In our series, most graft or anastomotic complications occurred during the initial period of our experience. Additionally, the duration of surgery also gradually decreased from 6 h to a little less than 4 h with increasing experience. Une *et al* similarly reported a significant reduction in operative time from 275 to 215 min ($p = 0.002$) after the first 25 cases [54]. It is advisable to acquire a large experience in performing conventional off-pump CABGs through a sternotomy approach and MIDCAB procedures before beginning with MICS-CABG surgery.

## 5.8   Results

We had the opportunity to further evolve the previously established technique of MICS-CABG procedures by developing a method of performing this operation with BITAs through a left anterolateral mini-thoracotomy for selected patients. This was chiefly possible due to the vast experience of off-pump CABG [27] and MIDCAB surgery [29] that already existed in our institution. Our experience demonstrates that off-pump MICS-CABG with BITAs can be performed safely with very good procedural outcomes that are comparable to those achieved through a median sternotomy [28]. Briefly, none of the 88 patients in our series required intraoperative conversions to CPB or sternotomy. A total of 209 distal anastomoses (mean $2.4 \pm 0.5$) were performed, with 57 patients undergoing double, 29 triple and 2 quadruple CABG. There was no in-hospital mortality and five patients underwent re-exploration for bleeding. No patient developed stroke or chest wound infections. Other groups have reported an early mortality ranging between 0% and 1.6% for patients undergoing MICS-CABG [5, 6, 7, 36, 37]. Comparing MICS-CABG series with studies involving conventional CABG would not be entirely appropriate on the one hand due to the inclusion of the learning curves of operating surgeons performing the MICS-CABG procedures and on the other due to the inclusion of only highly selected low-risk patients in the MICS-CABG studies, which is not usually the case in studies concerning conventional CABG. Nevertheless, a rough comparison would at least raise an alarm if the results of this operation were much worse than contemporary series reporting results of conventional CABG. The reported early mortality of MICS-CABG is comparable to that observed in the on-pump group in the Randomized On/Off Bypass (ROOBY) (1.3%) [35] and the Arterial Revascularization Trials (ART) (1.4%) [44]. Early mortality after MICS-CABG is even less than half of 2.5% observed in the international CABG Off- or On-Pump Revascularization Study (CORONARY) [33]. The results of our MICS-CABG series match well with our recently reported outcomes in almost 1200 patients undergoing off-pump CABG with BITAs (30-day mortality: 0.7%) [27].

An important factor that influences short and long-term outcomes following CABG is the completeness of revascularization [55], which was addressed previously. Therefore, it is important to again emphasize that the suitability of the coronary anatomy for achieving complete revascularization through a MICS-CABG procedure should be one of the most important criteria for patient selection and should be left to the discretion of the operating surgeon based on his/her experience and comfort level.

## 5.9    Future Perspectives

MICS-CABG can be effectively performed with very low postoperative complication rates and very good angiographic outcomes, thus, promising good long-term results in well selected patients. BITA grafting can be utilized without the concern of developing sternal wound complications. Left coronary total arterial revascularization with this approach and PCI of the right coronary system could potentially revolutionize hybrid coronary revascularization in the future. A multidisciplinary "heart team" approach is necessary for this purpose. However, for widespread acceptance worldwide, this procedure requires simplification to make it more reproducible and more evidence supporting it needs to be generated. Indications and selection criteria should be well-defined. Finally, the aim of MICS should be a total endoscopic/robot-assisted procedure performed with automated, but reliable anastomotic connectors without the use of rib-spreading.

# References

1. Chang C, Raza S, Altarabsheh SE, Delozier S, Sharma UM, Zia A, et al. Minimally invasive approaches to surgical aortic valve replacement: a meta-analysis. Ann Thorac Surg. 2018;106:1881–9.
2. Davierwala PM, Seeburger J, Pfannmueller B, Garbade J, Misfeld M, Borger MA, et al. Minimally invasive mitral valve surgery: "the Leipzig experience". Ann Cardiothorac Surg. 2013;2:744–50.
3. Diegeler A, Spyrantis N, Matin M, Falk V, Hambrecht R, Autschbach R, et al. The revival of surgical treatment for isolated proximal high grade LAD lesions by minimally invasive coronary artery bypass grafting. Eur J Cardiothorac Surg. 2000;17:501–4.
4. Cuartas MM, Javadikasgari H, Pfannmueller B, Seeburger J, Gillinov AM, Suri RM, Borger MA. Mitral valve repair: robotic and other minimally invasive approaches. Prog Cardiovasc Dis. 2017;60:394. https://doi.org/10.1016/j.pcad.2017.11.002.
5. Kikuchi K, Chen X, Mori M, et al. Perioperative outcomes of off-pump minimally invasive coronary artery bypass grafting with bilateral internal thoracic arteries under direct visiondagger. Interact Cardiovasc Thorac Surg. 2017;24:696–701.
6. Mcginn JT Jr, Usman S, Lapierre H, et al. Minimally invasive coronary artery bypass grafting: dual-center experience in 450 consecutive patients. Circulation. 2009;120(11 Suppl):S78–84.
7. Nambiar P, Kumar S, Mittal CM, Saksena K. Minimally invasive coronary artery bypass grafting with bilateral internal thoracic

arteries: will this be the future? J Thorac Cardiovasc Surg. 2018;155:190–7.

8. Calafiore AM, Di Mauro M, Teodori G, Di Giammarco G, Cirmeni S, Contini M, et al. Impact of aortic manipulation on incidence of cerebrovascular accidents after surgical myocardial revascularization. Ann Thorac Surg. 2002;73:1387–93.

9. Cohn LH, Adams DH, Couper GS, et al. Minimally invasive cardiac valve surgery improves patient satisfaction while reducing costs of cardiac valve replacement and repair. Ann Surg. 1997;226:421–6. 428.

10. Gammie JS, Zhao Y, Peterson ED, et al. J. Maxwell Chamberlain Memorial Paper for adult cardiac surgery. Less-invasive mitral valve operations: trends and outcomes from the Society of Thoracic Surgeons Adult Cardiac Surgery Database. Ann Thorac Surg. 2010;90(5):1401–8, 1410.e1; discussion 1408-10. https://doi.org/10.1016/j.athoracsur.2010.05.055.

11. Iribarne A, Easterwood R, Russo MJ, et al. A minimally invasive approach is more cost-effective than a traditional sternotomy approach for mitral valve surgery. J Thorac Cardiovasc Surg. 2011;142(6):1507–14. https://doi.org/10.1016/j.jtcvs.2011.04.038. Epub 2011 Jun 14.

12. Von Oppell UO, Mohr FW. Chordal replacement for both minimally invasive and conventional mitral valve surgery using premeasured Gore-Tex loops. Ann Thorac Surg. 2000;70(6):2166–8.

13. Carpentier A, Loulmet D, Aupecle B, et al. Computer assisted open heart surgery. First case operated on with success. C R Acad Sci III. 1998;321:437–42.

14. Carpentier A, Loulmet D, et al. Open heart operation under video surgery and minithoracotomy. First case ( mitral valvuloplasty) operated with sucess. C R Acad Sci III. 1996;319:219–23.

15. Falk V, Walther T, Autschbach R, et al. Robot-assisted minimally invasive solo mitral valve operation. J Thorac Cardiovasc Surg. 1998;115(2):470–1.

16. Casselman FP, Van Slycke S, Wellens F, et al. Mitral valve surgery can now routinely be performed endoscopically. Circulation. 2003;108(Suppl 1):II48–54.

17. Gillinov AM, Mihaljevic T, Javadikasgari H, et al. Early results of robotically assisted mitral valve surgery: analysis of the first 1,000 cases. J Thorac Cardiovasc Surg. 2018;155:82.

18. Mcclure RS, Athanasopoulos LV, Mcgurk S, et al. One thousand minimally invasive mitral valve operations: early outcomes, late

outcomes, and echocardiographic follow-up. J Thorac Cardiovasc Surg. 2013;145:1199–206.

19. Mohr FW, Falk V, Diegeler A, et al. Minimally invasive port-access mitral valve surgery. J Thorac Cardiovasc Surg. 1998;115(3):567–74, discussion 574–576.

20. Benetti FJ, Ballester C, Barnia A. Uso de la toracoscopia en cirugia coronaria para diseccion de la mamaria izquierda. Prensa Med Argent. 1994;81:877–9.

21. Borst C, Santamore WP, Smedira NG, et al. Minimally invasive coronary artery bypass grafting: on the beating heart and via limited access. Ann Thorac Surg. 1997;63(6 Suppl):S1–5.

22. Calafiore AM, Angelini GD. Left anterior small thoracotomy (LAST) for coronary artery revascularisation. Lancet. 1996;347:263–4.

23. Calafiore AM, Di Giammarco G, Teodori G, et al. Left anterior descending coronary artery grafting via left anterior small thoracotomy without cardiopulmonary bypass. Ann Thorac Surg. 1996;61:1658–65.

24. Reichenspurner H, Gulielmos V, Daniel WG, et al. Minimally invasive coronary-artery bypass surgery. N Engl J Med. 1997;336:67–8.

25. Angelini G, Wilde P, Salerno T, et al. Integrated left small thoracotomy and angioplasty for multivessel coronary artery revascularisation. Lancet. 1996;347:757–8.

26. Babliak O, Demianenko V, Melnyk Y, Revenko K, Pidgayna L, Stohov O. Complete coronary revascularization via left anterior thoracotomy. Innovations. 2019;14(4):330–41. https://doi.org/10.1177/1556984519849126. Epub 2019 May 20.

27. Davierwala PM, Leontyev S, Garbade J, Lehmann S, Holzhey D, Misfeld M, et al. Off-pump coronary artery bypass surgery with bilateral internal thoracic arteries: the Leipzig experience. Ann Cardiothorac Surg. 2018;7:483–91.

28. Davierwala PM, Verevkin A, Sgouropoulou SD, Hasheminejad E, Von Aspern K, Misfeld M, Borger MA. Minimally invasive coronary bypass surgery with bilateral internal thoracic arteries: early outcomes and angiographic patency. J Thorac Cardiovasc Surg. 2020. https://doi.org/10.1016/j.jtcvs.2019.12.136.

29. Holzhey DM, Cornely JP, Rastan AJ, Davierwala P, Mohr FW. Review of a 13-year single-center experience with minimally invasive direct coronary artery bypass as the primary surgical treatment of coronary artery disease. Heart Surg Forum. 2012;15:E61–8.

30. Nambiar P, Kumar S, Mittal CM, Sarkar IC. Outcomes of bilateral internal thoracic arteries in minimally invasive coronary artery bypass grafting with analogy to the SYNTAX trial. Innovations. 2019;14(3):227–35. https://doi.org/10.1177/1556984519837391.

31. Sakaguchi T, Mizuno T, Ryomoto M, Sekiya N, Totsugawa T, Tamura K, et al. A new multi-suction heart positioner for minimally invasive coronary artery bypass grafting. Ann Thorac Surg. 2019;109:e63. https://doi.org/10.1016/j.athoracsur.2019.07.068.

32. Roach GW, Kanchuger M, Mangano CM, Newman M, Nussmeier N, Wolman R, et al. Adverse cerebral outcome after coronary bypass surgery. N Engl J Med. 1996;335:1857–63.

33. Lamy A, Devereaux PJ, Prabhakaran D, Taggart DP, Hu S, Paolasso E, CORONARY Investigators, et al. Off-pump or on-pump coronary-artery bypass grafting at 30 days. N Engl J Med. 2012;366:1489–97.

34. Mack MJ, Head S, Holmes DR Jr, Ståhle E, Feldman TE, Colombo A, et al. Analysis of stroke occurring in the SYNTAX trial comparing coronary artery bypass surgery and percutaneous coronary intervention in the treatment of complex coronary artery disease. JACC Cardiovasc Interv. 2013;6:344–54.

35. Shroyer AL, Grover FL, Hattler B, Collins JF, Mcdonald GO, Kozora E, Veterans Affairs Randomized On/Off Bypass (ROOBY) Study Group, et al. On-pump versus off-pump coronary-artery bypass surgery. N Engl J Med. 2009;361:1827–37.

36. Rabindranauth P, Burns JG, Vessey TT, et al. Minimally invasive coronary artery bypass grafting is associated with improved clinical outcomes. Innovations. 2014;9:421–6.

37. Lemma M, Atanasiou T, Contino M. Minimally invasive cardiac surgery-coronary artery bypass graft. Multimed Man Cardiothorac Surg. 2013;2013:mmt007. https://doi.org/10.1093/mmcts/mmt007.

38. Goldstone AB, Atluri P, Szeto WY, et al. Minimally invasive approach provides at least equivalent results for surgical correction of mitral regurgitation: a propensity-matched comparison. J Thorac Cardiovasc Surg. 2013;145:748–56.

39. Kosmidou I, Chen S, Kappetein AP, Serruys PW, Gersh BJ, Puskas JD, et al. New-onset atrial fibrillation after PCI or CABG for left main disease: the EXCEL trial. J Am Coll Cardiol. 2018;71:739–48.

40. Kon ZN, Brown EN, Grant MC, Ozeki T, Burris NS, Collins MJ, et al. Warm ischemia provokes inflammation and regional hypercoagulability within the heart during off-pump coronary artery

bypass: a possible target for serine protease inhibition. Eur J Cardiothorac Surg. 2008;33:215–21.

41. Gaudino M, Benedetto U, Fremes S, et al. Radial-artery or saphenous-vein grafts in coronary-artery bypass surgery. N Engl J Med. 2018;378:2069–77.

42. Lytle BW, Blackstone EH, Sabik JF, Houghtaling P, Loop FD, Cosgrove DM. The effect of bilateral internal thoracic artery grafting on survival during 20 postoperative years. Ann Thorac Surg. 2004;78:2005–12.

43. Yi G, Shine B, Rehman SM, Altman DG, Taggart DP. Effect of bilateral internal mammary artery grafts on long-term survival: a meta-analysis approach. Circulation. 2014;130:539–45.

44. Taggart DP, Altman DG, Gray AM, Lees B, Nugara F, Yu LM, et al. Randomized trial to compare bilateral vs. single internal mammary coronary artery bypass grafting: 1-year results of the Arterial Revascularisation Trial (ART). Eur Heart J. 2010;31:2470–81.

45. Abdallah MS, Wang K, Magnuson EA, Spertus JA, Farkouh ME, Fuster V, FREEDOM Trial Investigators, et al. Quality of life after PCI vs CABG among patients with diabetes and multivessel coronary artery disease: a randomized clinical trial. JAMA. 2013;310:1581–90.

46. Head SJ, Mack MJ, Holmes DR Jr, Mohr FW, Morice MC, Serruys PW, et al. Incidence, predictors and outcomes of incomplete revascularization after percutaneous coronary intervention and coronary artery bypass grafting: a subgroup analysis of 3-year SYNTAX data. Eur J Cardiothorac Surg. 2012;41:535–41.

47. Cohen DJ, Van Hout B, Serruys PW, Mohr FW, Macaya C, Den Heijer P, et al. Synergy between PCI with taxus and cardiac surgery investigators. Quality of life after PCI with drug-eluting stents or coronary-artery bypass surgery. N Engl J Med. 2011;364:1016–26.

48. Lapierre H, Chan V, Sohmer B, et al. Minimally invasive coronary artery bypass grafting via a small thoracotomy versus off-pump: a case-matched study. Eur J Cardiothorac Surg. 2011;40:804–10.

49. Ziankou A, Ostrovsky Y. Early and midterm results of no-touch aorta multivessel small thoracotomy coronary artery bypass grafting: a propensity score-matched study. Innovations. 2015;10:258–67.

50. Guo MH, Wells GA, Glineur D, Fortier J, Davierwala PM, Kikuchi K, et al. Minimally Invasive coronary surgery compared

to STernotomy coronary artery bypass grafting: the MIST trial. Contemp Clin Trials. 2019;78:140–5.

51. Ruel M, Shariff MA, Lapierre H, et al. Results of the minimally invasive coronary artery bypass grafting angiographic patency study. J Thorac Cardiovasc Surg. 2014;147:203–8.

52. Valgimigli M, Bueno H, Byrne RA, Collet JP, Costa F, Jeppsson A, et al. 2017 ESC focused update on dual antiplatelet therapy in coronary artery disease developed in collaboration with EACTS. Eur J Cardiothorac Surg. 2018;53(1):34–78. https://doi.org/10.1093/ejcts/ezx334.

53. Felger JE, Chitwood WR, Nifong LW, Holbert D. Evolution of mitral valve surgery: toward a totally endoscopic approach. Ann Thorac Surg. 2001;72(4):1203–8; discussion 1208-9.

54. Une D, Lapierre H, Sohmer B, Rai V, Ruel M. Can minimally invasive coronary artery bypass grafting be initiated and practiced safely? A learning curve analysis. Innovations. 2013;8:403–9.

55. Omer S, Cornwell LD, Rosengart TK, Kelly RF, Ward HB, Holman WL, et al. Completeness of coronary revascularization and survival: impact of age and off-pump surgery. J Thorac Cardiovasc Surg. 2014;148:1307–15.